THE
CLEAR
SKIN
COOKBOOK

THE
CLEAR
SKIN
COOKBOOK

The vital vitamins and magic minerals you need for
smooth, blemish-free, younger-looking skin

DALE PINNOCK

SEVEN DIALS

CONTENTS

INTRODUCTION

I don't think there is anything that reflects a person's state of health more than their skin. Healthy people have wonderfully smooth glowing skin with even tone, and free from blemishes.

Also, it is true to say, there is nothing more distressing than angry red skin conditions, especially on areas of the body that are on display to the rest of the world, like the face and hands.

This is something that I know well from my own personal experience. Although, if I hadn't gone through that, I wouldn't be sitting here writing this today.

I'd love to tell you that there is some magical food or lifestyle that will eradicate skin problems or make your skin immune to any kind of upset, or prevent it from ageing. But, alas, this isn't the case. However, what I can certainly tell you is that diet and lifestyle have the potential to have a massive impact on the health

and functioning of the skin, the rate at which it ages, and the severity and healing time of skin lesions (acne spots, for example). This is what this book is about.

No matter what area of skin health you are concerned with, there is information here regarding potential nutritional links. Whether you are trying to tackle acne, you have stubborn eczema, or would just rather do the best you can to keep your skin looking young and healthy for as long as possible, then you are in the right place.

MY STORY

When I was 10 years old, my body started to change. I noticed a few little bumps on my chin but I wasn't overly concerned at first. The only thing that mattered to me in those days was being able to get down to the lake after school and at the weekends to do some fishing.

However, it was different a year later when I left junior school to go to secondary school. It was then that the trouble began. By this stage I was spotty. There's no other word for it. From forehead to chin, I was covered in nasty little red spots, a few bigger bumps and blackheads too. It didn't take long for everyone else in the class to notice this and I became the target of the usual names, such as Pizza Face and Zit Face.

Particularly at that stage in life, these things can make us very self-conscious and I became quite withdrawn, although I'd never let it show how much it affected me. By the time I reached the final year of school, it was a permanent preoccupation. I'd make a conscious effort to cover my face with a scarf, as I didn't want anyone to see my skin in daylight. Whenever I went into a shop I could never stand under the strip lighting because it would really show up my acne. I literally closed up and disappeared inside myself.

I went to doctor after doctor, specialist after specialist, and tried every conceivable lotion and potion they had to offer: strange sticky roll-on lotions, antibiotics, retinol gels, the works. Nothing whatsoever helped. One day, when I was about 15 or 16, a friend's mum lent me a book on nutrition and natural healthcare. I remember her telling me, 'Unless you look after what's going on inside, nothing will change on the outside.' Now, as a teenage boy, I wasn't immediately impressed with that advice!

However, I was so desperate that I read the book from cover to cover in a weekend. It changed my life: I gave up smoking, gave up eating meat, gave up most dairy products, and built a diet based on fruit, vegetables and whole grains, supplementing it with zinc, omega 3 and the B vitamins.

The changes were incredible. My skin certainly did clear. The red aggressive acne eventually disappeared, leaving not even the slightest mark. Beyond that, my body and mind were completely transformed and an entirely new person was born.

I have seen the powerful effect that food can have on our health first hand. It is simple yet profound. It was this experience that led me here today and has given me 100 per cent faith that if you implement the changes I recommend in this book, you too will start to see dramatic changes in the way your skin looks, not to mention the way that you feel inside.

WHAT THE SKIN DOES
AND HOW IT WORKS

If I were to ask you what the largest organ in the body is, I should imagine that many of you would say the brain, or the lungs, or the liver. Well, believe it or not, it's our skin. Many of us don't think of our skin as an organ, but it is the biggest organ of the human body, weighing an average of 2.7 kilograms.

KEY FUNCTIONS OF THE SKIN

The first major function of the skin is perhaps its most obvious, which is to act as a physical barrier to the outside world. All of our body's tissues are so delicate that even the most microscopic level of exposure to many external elements would be enough to kill us or cause severe damage and ill health. The skin offers us some degree of protection against this.

AN EXTENSION OF THE IMMUNE SYSTEM

The skin is a fully fledged part of our body's immune system. This is partially due to the physical barrier it provides, but there is more to it than that.

The skin is covered in billions of bacteria. Several types of bacteria live happily and symbiotically on its surface. One of the roles of these tiny passengers is defending us against certain types of potentially pathogenic bacteria. They can do this either through direct aggression towards the invader, or simply through competition for space on our skin's surface.

The skin can also help in the early stages of detection of a pathogen. There are cells embedded within the skin called Langerhans cells. These cells basically work as surveillance stations in the outer layers of the skin. They have the ability to detect specific pathogens and then communicate to our systemic immune system that trouble is coming.

TEMPERATURE REGULATION

The skin is a key player in regulating the temperature of the human body (thermoregulation). The surface of the skin is highly sensitive (more on this later), and as such can detect the slightest change in environmental temperature. It relays this information back to our brain's main control centre, the hypothalamus, which has a defined set point of what the body temperature should be. If internal or external factors cause the temperature to deviate outside this set point, the hypothalamus reacts by instigating the relevant responses to make the body warmer or cooler.

If we are too cold, the hypothalamus sends out nerve impulses, which cause the blood capillaries that supply the skin to narrow. This reduces heat loss through the surface of the skin, which is why we tend to look a little pale when we are cold. A signal is also sent to the skeletal muscles, which causes the body to shiver in order to generate heat.

When we are too hot, nerve impulses are sent to the skin, which cause the capillaries to dilate, allowing heat to escape through the skin's surface. The sweat glands are also stimulated and, as the sweat evaporates off the surface of the skin, it cools us down.

A SENSORY ORGAN

The skin is, of course, one of the major sensory organs, delivering the sense of touch. There are thousands of nerve endings within the skin, with some parts of the body (such as the fingertips) having higher concentrations than others. There are four main sensations that are transmitted through the skin: hot, cold, contact and pain.

There are a number of different types of pressure receptor that detect variations in touch, and allow us to determine textures, for example. The hairs on the skin also play a role in our sensory perception.

VITAMIN D PRODUCTION

One of the most exciting things that the skin does (well, for a nerd like me at least) is manufacture vitamin D upon exposure to ultraviolet rays from the sun. It does this by transforming cholesterol into vitamin D3, which is a precursor for the active form of this nutrient (it requires further conversion by the liver and kidneys). This transformation of cholesterol into vitamin D3 takes place in two deep areas of the skin: the stratum basale and the stratum spinosum.

THE STRUCTURE OF THE SKIN

The key to getting healthy skin is understanding its structure and the complexities of how it works.

THE EPIDERMIS

The epidermis is the outermost layer of the skin; its thickness varies throughout the body. On the soles of the feet and the palms of the hands, the epidermis is around 1–5mm thick. In contrast, the eyelids have an epidermis of 0.5mm. The epidermis is made up of five distinct layers. These are:

- The stratum corneum (the very top layer)
- The stratum lucidum
- The stratum granulosum
- The stratum spinosum
- The stratum basale (the very bottom layer)

Each layer is made up of different types of cells. The top layer, the stratum corneum, is made up of flat, dead skin cells that are shed, on average, every two weeks. The bottom layer, the stratum basale, is where new skin cells begin to form. Most of this layer is made up of cells that resemble columns, which push other growing cells upwards into the other layers of the skin, where they move through the ranks until they reach the stratum corneum, where they are eventually sloughed away.

There are also several types of specialist cell found within the epidermis. The first of these are the melanocytes. These are the cells responsible for giving our skin its pigment (melanin) and its lovely summer tan. They are located in the stratum basale, and secrete melanin in response to various stimuli, the main one being exposure to ultraviolet radiation. It's the melanin that gives colouration to the skin.

The next group of specialised cells in the epidermis are the Langerhans cells. These are involved in identifying potential pathogens, and sending signals to other branches of the immune system, as a kind of skin-bound early warning mechanism.

The final group of specialised cells in the epidermis are called Merkel cells, but strangely we are yet to discover exactly what they do!

THE DERMIS

The dermis is the next layer down in the skin's structure. It can be anywhere between 10 and 40 times thicker than the epidermis.

The very top part of the dermis is a rocky, bumpy terrain consisting of projections of protein fibres, blood vessels and nerve endings. The main type of cell that is found in the dermis is a cell called a fibroblast. The role of this busy cell is the constant manufacture and secretion of the two key structural components of the skin – collagen and elastin. These fibrous proteins give the skin its plumpness, firmness and elasticity. These cells are found mostly in the very upper layer of the dermis, in the region known as the dermal papillae.

The lower part of the dermal papillae is home to a series of microcapillaries. Some of these vessels are found lower down in the dermis too. Their role is to provide oxygen and nutrients to the epidermis, and also to regulate the skin's temperature.

Below the dermal papillae, the deeper parts of the dermis are known as the reticular dermis. This thick tissue, with many crisscrossing collagen and elastin fibres, is also home to the pilosebaceous unit. This structure consists of a hair, the hair follicle, a sebaceous gland and the musculature that makes the hair stand up or relax. It delivers lubrication to the skin in the form of sebum – the oily secretion released by the sebaceous gland. You will see later in the book that this can be the site of some problems. Sweat glands are also found in the reticular dermis, along with a series of ducts that carry sweat up to the epidermis during thermoregulation.

THE SUBCUTIS

The subcutis, often called the hypodermis, or subcutaneous layer, is the deepest and thickest part of the skin. This region is composed predominantly of collagen fibres and fat storage cells known as adipocytes. These fat cells are grouped together in clumps within the subcutis and not only offer a certain degree of cushioning to us, but can also work as an energy source. It is in this layer that we accumulate body fat, from sedentary living or over-consumption of the wrong types of foods, for example. Fats can be put back into circulation for fuel when we are following a weight-management diet or exercising effectively.

A high number of cells from the immune system, known as macrophages, are also found within the subcutis. These cells are able to identify any pathogens or dysfunctional cells within the body, and completely engulf them. Once they have engulfed them, they quickly break down the invader or damaged cell and remove it. This is a crude but effective first-line defence.

The subcutis is also home to some other larger structures. There is a series of thicker blood vessels which supply the smaller capillaries that run through the dermis. Bundled in with these is a series of lymphatic vessels that carry away any waste material from the epidermis and dermis, plus they can filter out some pathogenic material too.

The final group of structures housed in the subcutis are the nerves. Nervous tissue runs throughout the layers of the skin, with the nerve endings at the very top of the epidermis in order to allow us to touch and feel the world around us. The subcutis is where this nervous tissue begins to bundle together, plus there are some unique neurological structures that reside here, including the Pacinian corpuscle. This is actually a type of nerve receptor that detects pressure and vibration.

HOW THE SKIN AGES

The natural ageing of the skin is an inevitable process. I'm sorry to break that news to you. However, there is a lot that we can do to at least slow things down and make the best we can of the genes we've got. It is therefore important, now we are familiar with the skin's structure, to get an idea as to how it ages.

AGEING OF THE EPIDERMIS

One of the first things to occur in the ageing epidermis is a reduction in melanocytes. These are the cells that secrete colour pigment within the skin when we are exposed to ultraviolet radiation, as part of the skin's protective mechanism against radiation-mediated damage. As the number of melanocytes begins to decline, so does the protective pigment melanin. This, of course, puts the skin at greater risk of ultraviolet damage, which can lead to localised free radical formation (more on free radicals later), not to mention increasing susceptibility to skin cancer.

The immune cells known as Langerhans cells also start to decrease in number, which potentially reduces the barrier function of the skin against pathogens.

The main thing that people often notice as their skin ages is a dullness and change in colour and tone. This is largely due to the fact that the epidermis is losing nutrition as it ages.

Because this upper layer of the skin doesn't have its own blood supply, it gleans oxygen and nutrients from the dermis. As the skin ages, contact between the dermis and epidermis begins to diminish, and as such the delivery of these vital components reduces, which leads to poor cellular function. The end result is dull and lifeless skin.

The final assault on the epidermis is that it naturally begins to thin. This is because the rapid turnover of skin cells, described earlier, begins to slow down, and by our 70s it is 50 per cent less than in our 20s. This can make the skin look sunken and even saggy in places.

AGEING OF THE DERMIS

Ageing has a great effect on the dermis. The fibroblast cells that are responsible for the formation of collagen begin to shrivel, reducing the amount of collagen that is manufactured.

Existing collagen also begins to thin out, as there is a notable rise in enzymes called metalloproteinases that are responsible for breaking down collagen.

Remember that collagen and elastin, plus the extracellular matrix (the lattice-like mesh that helps give tissues structural support), are fundamental structures that enable the skin to maintain elasticity. Therefore the skin's youthful appearance begins to diminish.

The dermis is the area that houses most of the skin's blood supply. As we age there is a notable reduction in blood vessels, and therefore a reduction in circulation to this area. This will affect the amount of oxygen and nutrients that are delivered here. This is the main reason why ageing skin begins to look pale, and even feel colder – simply because there is less blood flow to the area.

These two processes lead to the density of the dermis decreasing notably during ageing.

AGEING OF THE SUBCUTANEOUS LAYER

This thick layer that consists mainly of fat cells and collagen fibres will also thin out. The number of fat cells will begin to reduce, giving less fullness to the skin. It will also affect thermoregulation, as natural insulation begins to reduce.

FACTORS INFLUENCING SKIN AGEING

THE FREE RADICAL THEORY OF AGEING

The most widely understood factor in the ageing of all tissues is free radical damage. Free radicals are highly reactive molecules that are produced during metabolic processes in the body. I won't go too deeply into free radicals at this point, as they are explained in greater detail in the antioxidants section on page 35 onwards.

Basically, they are chemically unbalanced molecules that are desperately seeking an electron to make them stable. They really aren't fussy blighters. They will nick one from anywhere. They collide into other molecules and steal electrons at any given opportunity. This causes damage to cells and tissues. Free radicals can also damage the DNA code of a cell, which will affect the way the cell reproduces. This can result in tissues slowly degrading. As tissues become more greatly affected in such a way, they are in essence ageing.

Some free radicals are produced naturally by the body during normal processes, whereas others are produced as the body deals with environmental factors – toxins from smoking, drinking excess alcohol and eating fried foods, as well as from pollution. Dealing with excessive free radicals involves certain lifestyle choices and a broad intake of antioxidants over a lifetime (see page 35 onwards for an in-depth look into this).

COLLAGEN CROSS LINKING

Our modern Western diet has a huge impact on the ageing of the skin as it's typically packed with refined carbohydrates and simple sugars: white rice, white bread, white pasta, fizzy drinks, ready meals and snack bars. Apart from this diet being devoid of nutrients and antioxidants, and being high in free-radical-forming components, it is also causing havoc to our blood sugar. In the body, these foods are quickly broken down into glucose, which rapidly enters our blood stream, dramatically elevating our blood sugar. The body's response to this is to release the hormone insulin, which encourages cells in the body to suck up this sugar, because if blood sugar levels remain high it can be life threatening.

Now, this process over time is linked to many lifestyle diseases, but that is beyond the subject matter of this book. What you need to know here is that when there is a sudden rise in blood sugar, the skin doesn't get away untouched.

A type of reaction takes place called a glycation reaction, which causes a rigid material to 'cross link' collagen and elastin fibres. This means the two are fused together in such a way that they lose their ability to stretch, essentially making them brittle. The skin loses its elasticity which can result in wrinkles and furrows.

The key to avoiding a rapid rise in blood sugar is to follow a low GI diet, which is a diet predominately made up of whole foods: unprocessed foods that provide an array of nutrients and which release their sugars into the bloodstream slowly and steadily. Whole foods are the type of foods recommended in this book!

GENERAL CONSIDERATIONS FOR THE MANAGEMENT OF SKIN DISORDERS

The conditions outlined below are the ones that are most responsive to dietary intervention. There are hundreds of different skin conditions, but not all will respond to dietary treatment. Those that require more specialised dermatological treatment have been omitted.

While each skin disorder has its own unique set of circumstances that require bespoke management, there are some dietary approaches that all of them will respond well to.

MANAGING INFLAMMATION

Most common skin conditions will involve active inflammation at varying stages of their progression. Inflammation is a necessary part of the healing process and something that shouldn't, and couldn't, be fully suppressed. It arises when changes have occurred in a tissue that may lead to damage or infection. Specific cells respond to this change by releasing chemical messengers that start the inflammatory process. These signals cause an increase in blood flow, causing redness and heat (known as rubor and calor), which increases the transport of oxygen, nutrients and immunological components, such as white blood cells, to the affected area. As the blood vessels widen to enhance circulation, the walls become slightly porous, which helps white blood cells move to the affected area with greater ease.

You can see how this is a necessary process for healing. However, it is this process that is responsible for the appearance of many skin lesions. Just think of the redness and heat of the early stages of an eczema flare-up, or the red anger of a newly formed acne spot. One of the keys to dietary management of skin conditions is to consume foods that help the body to reduce its inflammatory load. This could involve manipulating our intake of dietary fats, or focusing on groups of specific nutrients.

★ *Key foods for reducing inflammation:* omega 3 fatty acids – EPA and DHA, zinc.

IMPROVING THE BODY'S ABILITY TO FIGHT INFECTION

Fighting infection is important for two reasons. Firstly, in conditions such as acne, there is active infection within the skin itself. Assisting the body in its management of infection will help the lesions to clear more efficiently. The second reason is that in many skin conditions, the barrier properties of the skin can be compromised. Just think of eczema that is cracked or bleeding. This potentially allows for pathogens to get in. Keeping defences strong helps us to manage this. Thankfully there are some micronutrients that can influence white cell activity for example.

★ *Key nutrients/foods for fighting infection:* zinc, vitamin C, mushroom polysaccharides.

IMPROVING SKIN CELL FUNCTION

Another key area of managing skin conditions via dietary means is supplying the body with the necessary nutrients to improve the health of the skin cells, making the tissue function better as a whole. I know this sounds a little generic, but improving overall skin function can often be a better approach than trying to directly target specific physiological processes.

There are two main ways in which diet can influence skin tissue health. Firstly, it can influence the skin's ability to retain and utilise moisture. Providing adequate nutrients will keep cell membranes nicely fluid and supple.

Secondly, diet can regulate the rate of skin cell turnover. Several nutrients play a direct role in this. If the layers of the skin are being shed too slowly, it may contribute to the formation of blackheads (comedones); if they are shed too rapidly, it may lead to the scaling seen in psoriasis lesions. Providing the correct nutrients will help regulate the behaviour of skin cells.

★ *Key nutrients for keeping skin cells healthy:* omega 3, selenium, vitamin E.

VITAL VITAMINS

Vitamins are one of the most vital aspects of skincare and one that we should all make ourselves familiar with, if we want clear, vibrant skin.

However, most people have little idea what these little gems actually do for us, even in the general sense. If I were to ask, 'What exactly do vitamins do?', how many of us would be able to give a direct answer? Very few I should imagine. That is because we have been bombarded with huge amounts of media information about the next wonder vitamin, and how X vitamin may cause or cure Y condition.

Put as simply as possible, vitamins are facilitators of biochemical events in the body. There are millions of biochemical chain reactions happening in our bodies every second. Different metabolic processes change one compound into another, in order to allow it to undertake a certain function. Different chemical pathways process hormones, create communication chemicals that send messages between cells and tissues, process dietary substances – the list goes on. Virtually all of these processes will require vitamins in order for the chemical events to take place. So, it's clear to see that these are vital compounds; vitamin deficiency can cause serious illness.

It is a sad fact that the foods that dominate in the Western world of convenience and haste are often completely devoid of vitamins. They are commonly packed to the hilt with macronutrients such as fat, carbohydrate and protein, but micronutrients, such as vitamins and minerals, have been lost in the mass production process. As so many of us are consuming a Western diet, it's no wonder that skin problems are becoming more common.

The simplest way around this is to abandon the nasty ready meals that only require a few pricks from a fork and ten minutes being nuked in a microwave, and instead reach for fresh, wholesome, unadulterated ingredients. If this fills you with dismay, fear not. I will show you how affordable, easy and fun it is to prepare fresh foods for yourself.

Here's a brief outline of what does what when it comes to vitamins and your skin.

VITAMIN A

Vitamin A is one nutrient that has a long history of therapeutic use in skin conditions. There are two main forms of vitamin A: retinol and beta-carotene.

The retinoid form of this nutrient has been used by dermatologists in topical preparations for the treatment of conditions such as acne, lichen planus and psoriasis. These are all conditions that are associated with an increase in the production of keratin. This is a protein within the skin that, if produced to excess, can cause an increased turnover of skin cells and an increased risk of blocked pores. Vitamin A is also known to support skin structures, such as collagen, which can help to reduce excessive wrinkling of the skin.

Retinol is the animal form of vitamin A, and is found in abundance in foods such as red meat, liver, eggs and some cheeses.

Beta-carotene is the plant form of vitamin A, and is the pigment that gives bright orange foods their colour. Great examples of this are sweet potatoes, carrots, pumpkins and mangoes. Beta-carotene is a very potent fat-soluble antioxidant, so it can actually accumulate in the skin (see the antioxidant chapter for more details of this). This helps to provide a localised protection against free radical damage that can cause degradation of collagen fibres, which in the long term can lead to wrinkling and reduced fullness and youthfulness of the skin. An accumulation of beta-carotene in the skin also has an added benefit of delivering some localised anti-inflammatory activity, which can help to reduce the redness and physical appearance of skin lesions such as eczema flare-ups and acne breakouts. This anti-inflammatory effect is due to its antioxidant function. Several elements of the inflammatory process are triggered by localised free radical release from white blood cells in normal response to injury or infection, so adding some fat-soluble antioxidants to the mix is going to offer some protection against free radical-mediated inflammatory episodes.

★ *Best food sources:* eggs, liver, carrots, sweet potatoes, kale.

THE B VITAMINS

The B vitamins, as a group, are in my professional opinion one of the most important nutrients for skin health. The main emphasis of this book is on improving the skin's overall functioning as an organ from as many different angles as possible.

No other group of nutrients supports the skin in such a diverse way as the B vitamins. Each individual B vitamin affects different aspects of the skin's function and so together they allow for much healthier skin that can only look better as a result. Here is a breakdown of the many ways in which these nutrients can benefit the skin:

B1 (THIAMIN)

B1 is the nutrient to take if you want to give the skin a warm, healthy glow. This is because B1 supports microcirculation – the bed of tiny capillaries that deliver blood to the layers of the skin. By encouraging better microcirculation, we allow for a better supply of fresh oxygenated blood and nutrients, as well as more effective removal of waste materials, thus helping the skin to meet its metabolic needs to function more successfully. Plus improved circulation to the skin can give a nice glow.

★ *Best food sources:* asparagus, mushrooms, spinach, sunflower seeds, green peas, oats.

B2 (RIBOFLAVIN)

B2 doesn't particularly give any notable benefits when extra amounts are taken but a deficiency can leave your skin looking pretty grotty. When levels of this nutrient get too low, we see a dulling of the skin, along with patches of dryness. The most well-known symptom of B2 deficiency is angular stomatitis, which is a painful cracking in the corners of the mouth.

★ *Best food sources:* mushrooms, spinach, asparagus, broccoli, eggs.

B3 (NIACIN)

B3 is a valuable nutrient for skin health, both from a maintenance perspective as well as from a therapeutic one. Its main role is in oxygenating the skin. It does this by acting as a vasodilator for the dermal microcirculation, which means that it forces the tiny network of blood vessels to widen, causing an increase in circulation to the upper layers of the skin. This helps with a number of activities, from wound healing to cellular function.

A word of caution, however. Many people find that this nutrient can cause a rapid and sometimes uncomfortable flushing of the skin, creating patches of itchy redness. While this can be initially alarming, it is merely a demonstration that the nutrient is working. If you want a more subtle effect, you need to choose a different form of this nutrient. Commercially available niacin comes in two different chemical forms: nicotinic acid and niacinamide. The nicotinic acid form is the one that flushes the skin, whereas the niacinamide form delivers a much more gentle circulatory stimulation, without causing the pronounced flushing.

★ *Best food sources:* mushrooms, tuna, sea vegetables.

B5 (PANTOTHENIC ACID)

B5 is used most commonly for individuals going through periods of intense stress,

as it is involved in supporting the adrenal glands.

However, it does have some application in skin health. It has frequently been used for treating itchy inflamed skin lesions such as eczema and contact dermatitis.

★ *Best food sources:* mushrooms, cauliflower, sunflower seeds, tomatoes, strawberries.

B6 (PYRIDOXINE)

B6 is an incredibly useful nutrient for the more aesthetic end of the skincare spectrum. It is closely involved in regulating the balance of sodium and potassium. As such, it has proved very helpful for managing fluid accumulation in tissues, which makes it a useful nutrient to bear in mind for issues such as puffy eyes and a puffy face.

★ *Best food sources:* spinach, (bell) peppers, garlic, tuna, cauliflower, banana, celery, Brussels sprouts.

B12 (CYANOCOBALAMIN)

B12 is predominantly used in the body for red blood cell formation. This can aid in oxygen transportation, and therefore it can help give the skin a healthy glow. While not directly therapeutic, it is certainly a useful aid for making the skin look a little better.

★ *Best food sources:* liver, red snapper, prawns (shrimps), salmon, kelp, spirulina, tempeh, miso.

VITAMIN C

Vitamin C has often been portrayed as a universal cure-all that has benefits for almost every conceivable ailment.

It plays a vital role in the manufacture of collagen so, from a long-term perspective, it can be a useful nutrient to support a healthy ageing process, including the ageing of the skin.

Collagen, the most abundant protein in the body, makes up about 25 per cent of all proteins in the body. Its primary roles are to maintain the strength and elasticity of connective tissues, and to enable tissues, including the skin, to hold their structure. It is the job of vitamin C to link different parts of the collagen molecule together as it is being constructed, so sufficient vitamin C intake can aid in the adequate manufacture of collagen.

★ *Best food sources:* citrus fruit, goji berries, spinach, red (bell) peppers.

VITAMIN D

Vitamin D has become one of the most talked about nutrients of modern times. Barely a week goes by without it appearing in the world's press. There have been huge leaps in research that have highlighted the protective role that vitamin D plays in many lifestyle diseases. There is also some evidence to suggest that vitamin D may be useful in the treatment and management of psoriasis.

Skin cells have receptors for the active form of vitamin D (after it has been converted in the body), and vitamin D regulates the turnover of skin cells. As psoriasis is an over-accelerated turnover of skin cells, extra intake of this nutrient may well prove beneficial.

★ *Best food sources:* mushrooms, cheese, fish.

VITAMIN E

Vitamin E is probably the most famous 'skin nutrient'. It is a very well-known antioxidant, with particular relevance to skin health. As it is fat-soluble, it can move into the fatty layers of the skin where it can offer maximum protection from free radicals. In these layers there is a large proportion of collagen, which gives the skin its structural integrity. The collagen here is susceptible to attack from free radicals, which in time can lead to wrinkling, dulled appearance of the skin, and a slower healing time for skin lesions. It will also make the skin look less plump.

There is another potential way that vitamin E is useful for the management of skin conditions, which is by supporting the immune system. In issues such as acne, for example, there is an infectious element and it is vital that we have a strong, healthy immune system that is able to deal with the infection quickly and efficiently. Vitamin E protects the thymus gland, which is one of the main tissues involved in manufacturing leukocytes (white blood cells) and can also protect leukocytes from damage during oxidative stress.

★ *Best food sources:* avocados, nuts, olive oil.

FOOD PREPARATION FOR MAXIMUM VITAMIN INTAKE

It's all well and good reaching for higher-quality ingredients and fresh foods, but if they are cooked in the wrong way, or cooked to death, then much of the benefit that you hope to gain will sadly be lost. There are some simple rules to cooking fresh vegetables that will retain as much of their goodness as possible.

Most of the beneficial vitamins described above are in fact water-soluble substances. If you follow that age-old British tradition of boiling vegetables to within an inch of their lives, then you may as well throw the veggies away and just drink the water. That's where all of the nutrients will be! As the nutrients are water-soluble, they will naturally want to leach out of the food and into the water. If you boil the water, this process will accelerate drastically, and if you leave the veggies in for too long, they will become lifeless and gloopy and taste of nothing.

The cooking methods I favour are steaming and sautéing. Both retain most of the water-soluble nutrients (vitamin C, the B vitamins) in the food. Sautéing especially brings the flavours of the food to life.

THE MAGIC OF MINERALS

Minerals have to be the forgotten allies in the world of nutrition. This is especially true when it comes to skincare. Virtually everyone is familiar with the concept of calcium for healthy bones and iron for energy. But how often do we consider minerals when we think of skin health? Certain minerals and trace minerals have a huge role to play in both maintaining the day-to-day health of the skin, and also delivering a therapeutic benefit when tackling active skin conditions.

CHROMIUM

Chromium is one mineral that may not immediately spring to mind when it comes to looking after the health of the skin. However, there is an indirect but vital link. One of the most destructive influences on the health of the skin over a lifetime and the rate of skin ageing is continual blood sugar spikes. In our modern world of convenience and pro-cessed foods, we are consuming huge amounts of high glycaemic foods, such as white bread, white rice, white pasta, sugary drinks and snacks. This means we are eating foods that release their sugars into our bloodstream very fast. This gives us a quick energy boost, but our blood sugar is not meant to rise rapidly. We are designed to be eating whole foods such as fruits, vegetables, nuts and seeds. These foods release their sugars slowly and steadily. It's dangerous for our blood sugar to rise too rapidly, and because of this we have an effective way of dealing with it.

When our blood sugar rises, insulin is released from the pancreas. Insulin communicates to cells in our body, telling them to take in sugar from the blood and convert it into energy. The faster our blood sugar rises, the greater the release of insulin. However, the insulin system can only deal with so much sugar at one time.

Once we have passed the system's capacity to deal with any more sugar, the body turns it into fat. It can also be deposited in other tissues and this is when trouble can start for the health of our skin. If excess sugar reaches the dermis, it can very quickly start to bond with collagen and elastin, in a process called glycation. Once the sugar has formed a permanent bond with collagen and elastin, it becomes an advanced glycation end product or AGE (which is rather appropriate). AGEs can then form further bonds with collagen and elastin, creating cross links between fibres. This causes the collagen lattice to become stiff, rather than supple, which in turn leads to a loss in youthful skin elasticity, speeding up the ageing of the skin.

So, where does chromium fit into all of this? Well, chromium is used by the body to create something called glucose tolerance factor (GTF). This molecule is involved in stabilising blood sugar levels by working alongside insulin to further enhance a cell's ability to take in glucose (sugar) effectively. It will help blood sugar to stay at a safe level for longer, which has a myriad of health benefits, but where the skin is concerned it means that there will be less likelihood that sugar will become deposited in the collagen matrix to form AGEs.

★ *Best food sources:* yeast, oysters, whole grains, potatoes.

SELENIUM

Selenium is a mineral that has been talked about a lot in recent years, and one that is still deficient in the Western diet.

It is a trace mineral, and as such is only required in tiny amounts, yet many of us still fail to consume enough. Part of this is because of the poor quality of the soil due to today's farming methods. The more intensely land is farmed, the more its natural mineral content begins to decline. As the nutritional composition of fresh produce is a reflection of the soil in which it is grown, a lot of food today is lower in micronutrients than it was even 10 years ago. Couple this with poor food choices, and you soon see why our intake of certain nutrients has declined to such an extent.

Selenium is a key player in long-term skin health. This is mostly due to its potent antioxidant-promoting activity. Selenium is a cofactor (a substance necessary for the formation of another substance) in the production of a very powerful antioxidant enzyme called glutathione peroxidase (GP). GP plays a vital role in protecting cells and tissues from biochemical damage caused by free radicals. It can offer protection both to skin cells and also to the matrix of collagen fibres that offer support and structure to our skin. If these fibres become damaged, from free radical attack, or cross-linking due to high blood glucose, it can leave our skin looking dull and shallow, and make us much more susceptible to wrinkling earlier in life.

The other benefit of selenium is that it will deliver a certain amount of anti-inflammatory activity. This is again due to its antioxidant action. When a skin lesion, such as an acne spot or an eczema flare-up is red and angry, that means there is a lot of active localised inflammation. Part of the inflammatory response is enhanced by localised free radical release (there are many steps involved in activating inflammation). Adding additional antioxidant nutrients and precursors can offer some benefit in the reduction of redness and severity of inflammatory lesions.

★ *Best food sources:* Brazil nuts, shiitake mushrooms, prawns (shrimps), salmon, tuna, sunflower seeds.

SILICA

This wonderful mineral is one of the most important for long-term skin health, yet one which is seldom talked about outside of the health food world. Silica is found in a wide variety of fruits and vegetables. Its presence in a food often gives it a smooth, shiny skin. Think about a red (bell) pepper or a cucumber. That shiny skin on the outside is due to the high levels of silica present.

Silica is known to activate certain enzymes that are involved in the production of collagen. While the turnover of collagen is extremely slow, it is vital that we do all we can to ensure that the production of high-quality collagen is carried out as best as is physically possible for our body.

★ *Best food sources:* cucumbers, (bell) peppers, leeks, green beans.

SULPHUR

Organic sulphur is one of the most important nutrients to the long-term beauty, structure and ageing of the skin. It is the most broadly used mineral in both the production and maintenance of the extra-cellular matrix – the lattice-like mesh that helps give tissues structural support. The main component of this matrix is a group of proteins called proteoglycans, which bind to collagen within the matrix to form this vast web of supportive material. Sulphur is a key component of these proteins and therefore ensuring an adequate sulphur intake is essential for a healthy appearance to the skin.

★ *Best food sources:* onions, garlic, leeks, eggs, fish.

ZINC

Zinc is one of the single most important nutrients for skin health.

Male and female, young and old, will all benefit from an adequate intake of this nutrient.

Zinc is involved in the production and regulation of over 200 hormones, including powerful ones such as testosterone.

Testosterone is the main hormone involved in instigating acne lesions. Testosterone, when converted into the aggressive form (dihydrotestosterone), can have a stimulatory effect upon the sebaceous glands. It causes them to start producing larger than necessary amounts of sebum. It also causes the sebum to become slightly thicker and more viscous. This increase in thicker sebum creates an environment more conducive to the formation of comedones (blackheads). These are formed when sebum combines with keratin to make a thick sticky plug that blocks a hair follicle. This plug works like fly paper, trapping bacteria that normally live happily on the surface of the skin. These staphylococcus bacteria begin to accumulate in the sebum/keratin plug, and are able to instigate infection. There is then an active infection within the hair follicle, and an acne spot is born.

By increasing our intake of zinc, the behaviour of testosterone can be kept in check and its effect upon sebaceous glands is far less aggressive.

Zinc has a further regulatory effect upon sebaceous glands, separate from that of hormonal control. It has the ability to help regulate the sebaceous glands. If the skin is too oily, zinc seems to have the ability to reduce the secretion of sebum. If the skin is very dry, zinc seems to be able to increase the secretion of sebum to normalise the oil content of the skin.

Zinc is also involved in the coding of genes within key white blood cells that regulate the way in which these cells respond to infection. This will help support the management of bacterial infection.

★ *Best food sources:* shellfish, pumpkin seeds, mushrooms, spinach.

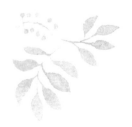

AMAZING ANTIOXIDANTS

Unless you have been inhabiting a different planet for the last 20 years, you will have heard of antioxidants. These seemingly mysterious compounds have become a fashionable buzz word, and it is almost impossible to pick up a glossy magazine without seeing at least one reference to them. There is a great deal of hype surrounding antioxidants, but never have they been more misunderstood.

WHAT IS AN ANTIOXIDANT?

There is a constant battle taking place in our bodies. Every cell has the ability to create its own energy supply – a molecule called ATP – by metabolising glucose from the food we eat. This is what keeps every cell alive, and is referred to as cellular respiration. During this process, a series of mischievous compounds, known as 'free radicals', is formed. Now, I know that their name makes them sound like some extreme guerilla military group, but they are in fact metabolic by-products that are chemically unbalanced.

Without getting too geeky, different chemical elements require a certain amount of electrons to be present within their outer structure in order to be 'stable'. If they don't have sufficient electrons, they will desperately seek a spare electron. An 'unstable' molecule will smash into unsuspecting 'stable' molecules, trying to steal one. When this occurs, the attacked molecule itself becomes unstable, beginning a chain reaction. This cascade can eventually damage the genetic material within a cell, which can then lead to the cell function-ing poorly, or even affect the way in which the cell behaves when it divides.

In light of this, there is a huge link between free radicals and the onset of cancers, and certainly the ageing of body tissues.

But, it's not all doom and gloom. The body actually produces its own free rad-ical compounds that are of benefit to us in certain situations. The immune system is a prime example of this. Certain types of white blood cells secrete free radicals in order to assist in the inflammatory response when the body has been injured or is coming under attack from an infec-tious agent. However, not allowing these natural free radicals to get out of control is a valuable key to symptomatic manage-ment of many different conditions and ailments.

Free radicals are also formed when our body has to metabolise toxic compounds to remove them from the body, such as those from smoking, drinking too much alcohol, environmental pollutants and certain nasty dietary compounds. The free radicals produced from the metabolis-ation of such environmental compounds are far more abundant and aggressive than those formed by normal cellular pro-cesses. That is why these sorts of toxins are so closely associated with premature ageing.

Antioxidants are a natural solution to the electron problem faced by free radicals. By their very nature, antioxidants are electron donors. They can donate an electron to the panicking free radical, thus disarming it and stopping it from causing trouble by damaging other molecules in its quest for stability. However, once an antioxidant has donated an electron to a free radical, it then becomes a free radical itself.

Nature is a wonderful thing. When we consume foods that are naturally rich in antioxidants, we also consume a whole host of other active phytochemicals that help to recycle the antioxidants once they have donated their electron. Often you will find that antioxidant-rich foods contain several types of antioxidant, each with the ability to recycle one another.

A word of warning: while it can be very useful to supplement with antioxidant nutrients to support our health, it is always wise to look for a product that contains a whole range of different antioxidants. This way you can ensure that there are sufficient supportive compounds present for adequate recycling, once the antioxidant has donated its electron.

There is now a large amount of evidence showing the negative effects of taking high doses of individual antioxidant nutrients in isolation – such as taking large doses of beta-carotene.

This is because taking an individual antioxidant without all the other supportive compounds to recycle it, can in fact increase our free radical load and create more problems.

THE SOLUBILITY ISSUE

If, like me, you have tried virtually every single skincare brand on the market, you will have noticed that many products these days have 'added antioxidants' to increase the antioxidant profile of the product. You may also be aware of many of the nutritional supplements aimed at skin health that seem to list endless antioxidants. This all sounds wonderful, but unfortunately it means that all antioxidants have been bunched together and it's assumed that they all do exactly the same thing. There are literally hundreds of compounds in the plant kingdom that can work as antioxidants in the body. It really stands to reason that the behaviour of these compounds will be as diverse as the array of antioxidants themselves. Therefore it shouldn't be assumed that all antioxidants will do the same thing, be active in the same parts of the body, and be distributed in the body in similar ways.

Broadly speaking, antioxidants can be split into two main groups: water-soluble antioxidants and fat-soluble antioxidants.

WATER-SOLUBLE ANTIOXIDANTS

Water-soluble antioxidants, as the name suggests, are water-soluble compounds. This means that they can happily be absorbed through the gut wall but will then mainly deliver their benefits within the systemic circulation. Therefore, they will offer great protection to the lining of blood vessels, as well as to some areas of the liver and kidneys, for example. This type of antioxidant doesn't stay in the body very long, and is rapidly excreted via the kidneys. Water-soluble antioxidants include vitamin C and flavonoids, a group of phytochemicals.

FAT-SOLUBLE ANTIOXIDANTS

Fat-soluble antioxidants, on the other hand, will behave slightly differently. They will not stay in systemic circulation for long because they will naturally seek a fat-rich environment. They will rapidly migrate into fatty tissues, such as the eyes and, of course, the fatty subcutaneous layer of the skin. When they move into these tissues, they generally stay there until they are fully spent and broken down, as there is no mechanism that can pull them out of fatty tissues back into circulation. As such, they are present in the body for much longer than water-soluble antioxidants and can begin to accumulate and deliver their effects for a much longer period of time. Fat-soluble antioxidants include vitamin A, vitamin E and the carotenoids (which include beta-carotene, alpha-carotene, astaxanthin and lycopene).

It is the fat-soluble antioxidants that are of greatest interest in the context of skin health. It is in the fatty layer of the skin that the collagen matrix, the lattice-like structure that gives skin its structural support, is found. This collagen matrix can frequently come under free radical attack from a whole host of different environmental influences. Therefore we need to supply adequate antioxidant protection in order to prevent or reduce the extent of any damage that may occur.

Damage to the collagen matrix can cause wrinkles, and cause the skin to sag and lose elasticity (just think of the wrinkled mouth of a long-term smoker). Fat-soluble antioxidants, such as the carotenoids can offer this protection. When they move into the subcutaneous layer, they quickly accumulate and can lie in waiting for any opportunistic free radicals, ready to disarm them before they can cause any damage. To ensure that we have adequate levels of fat-soluble antioxidants present at all times to offer this protection, it is vital that we consume foods that are naturally rich in them every day.

It is worth mentioning here that we also need to ensure that we consume these foods with a good-quality fat source. This simple combination will ensure that the fat-soluble antioxidants get taken up much more effectively in the digestive tract. This can be as simple as creating a tomato and red bell pepper salad, with an olive oil-based dressing. The tomatoes and peppers are dense sources of carotenoids and the addition of the olive oil increases their solubility, and gives an ideal transport vehicle to carry these wonderful antioxidants across the gut wall.

It also stands to reason that we should follow a diet and lifestyle that minimises the production of free radicals in the body. It is impossible to avoid them completely, as their formation is a normal part of metabolic activity. However, certain foods and lifestyle choices can cause a huge surge in free radical production. Smoking is a perfect example of this. Excessive alcohol intake and consuming too much fried food and overly processed food also cause a massive increase in free radical production. So, you guessed it, the key to long-term skin health is don't smoke, keep the booze to a minimum, and consume a diet that is predominantly fresh, wholefood-based and rich in the types of foods outlined in this book.

FACE FATS

We seem to have become completely obsessed with fat. Low-fat this, reduced-fat that. It has become a demonized nutrient. In some cases, it is certainly wise to reduce our fat intake. Saturated animal fats, such as those found in red meat, can trigger inflammatory issues in the body, which can be damaging to the heart, the circulatory system and the joints, and can even worsen some skin lesions like eczema and psoriasis. However, the trend that most health-conscious people take is to go 'low-fat' on almost everything, and this can be detrimental to many aspects of our health.

Fats are a vital nutrient for our body. Virtually every single hormone in the body is manufactured from fat. This includes oestrogen and testosterone. Fats are also the key materials used for the creation of different communication molecules, and structural components necessary for normal day-to-day functioning of the body. They also provide the source material for the manufacture of nutrients. So, as you can imagine, cutting them out completely can be bad for long-term health.

The key is to make sure that you choose the right types of fat, and that you're not guzzling down pizza and chips every night. The emphasis should be on unsaturated fats such as those found in nuts and seeds, oily fish, avocados and olive oil.

OMEGA 3 FATTY ACIDS

Unless you have been living in a cave, or have distanced yourself from all forms of communication in the last decade, chances are you have heard a lot about omega 3 and the myriad benefits that it delivers. Omega 3 is an essential fatty acid most commonly found in oily fish, some nuts, such as walnuts, and some seeds, such as flax and hemp. It is a vital yet widely deficient nutrient.

ANTI-INFLAMMATORY ACTION

Omega 3 fatty acids are one of the most important tools that we have at our disposal for the treatment of any type of inflammatory issue. When we process and metabolise dietary fats, one of the metabolic end products is a group of communication molecules known as prostaglandins. One of the main roles of the prostaglandins is to regulate different aspects of the inflammatory response. There are three different types of prostaglandin: series 1, series 2 and series 3. Series 1 and series 3 are involved in dampening down and deactivating the inflammatory response. Series 2 prostaglandins, in contrast, are involved in the instigation of the inflammatory response, and can make any currently active inflammation worse.

The type of prostaglandins produced will depend on the type of dietary fat that is consumed. For example, saturated animal fats are very high in a fatty acid called arachidonic acid, which, when metabolised, causes a rise in series 2 prostaglandins – the ones responsible for exacerbating inflammation. Oily fish, however, is high in omega 3 fatty acids, which, when metabolised, will cause an increase in the production of series 1 and series 3 prostaglandins – the ones that tackle inflammation. So, in essence, manipulating our dietary fat intake can directly influence the inflammatory response in our body.

Remember that virtually all skin lesions involve inflammation. The red, itchy flare-ups of eczema and the painful swelling of acne are all signs of active inflammation. So, any techniques we can adopt to make this less severe are of huge importance.

CELL MEMBRANE HEALTH

Every cell in our body has a fatty membrane that gives the cell its shape, keeps the cell contents in, and keeps toxins and pathogens out. Cell membranes are made of a double layer of molecules called phospholipids, which are composed of fatty acids. The cell membranes also house a whole array of different receptors and transporters. These complex and highly organised structures allow interactions between the inner workings of the cell and its outer environment. They allow hormones to bind to the cell and instigate changes to the way in which the cell behaves. They allow nutrients to successfully enter the cell, and for waste material to be removed. A healthy membrane means a healthy cell, which means healthy tissues.

Cell membranes require a constant stream of fatty acids in order to be able to maintain themselves, to ensure that they remain soft, supple and strong, and that their many receptor sites remain fully functional. As you have probably guessed by now, the fats required for this maintenance are the omega 3 fatty acids.

If the membranes of skin cells are working optimally, the skin as an organ will function much better. There will be better oxygen delivery, better transport of nutrients to the tissue, and also the skin's ability to retain moisture will be greatly improved.

There is another added plus point. As the skin starts to behave better as an organ, the effects of any topical products that we use on our skin, such as moisturisers and face masks, will be greatly enhanced.

OMEGA 6 FATTY ACIDS

The other essential fatty acid is the omega 6 fatty acid.

This is found in the highest concentrations in seed oils.

HANGING IN THE BALANCE

Omega 6 fatty acids have some vitally important functions in the body. When converted in the right way, they can also deliver some anti-inflammatory effects, which have been well documented in cases of eczema and acne.

However, there are issues surrounding

omega 6 fatty acids, mainly around the way in which they convert during their metabolism. Omega 6 can, when consumed in levels beyond daily requirements, be converted into series 2 prostaglandins – the ones that activate and exacerbate inflammation. They can also be converted into another inflammatory stimulator – lipoxygenase. In addition, there is new evidence emerging that some by-products of omega 6 fatty acids are found in all acne lesions, and are believed to be part of the instigation process of this condition.

BALANCING ACT

The key to ensuring that the omega 3 and omega 6 essential fatty acids deliver the anti-inflammatory benefits described above is ensuring we have the right balance of them in our diet. We need a ratio of 2:1, in favour of omega 3. That's twice as much omega 3 as omega 6. However, for many in the Western world, this ratio is completely reversed. This has led to devastating patterns of disease. There are now links between excessive omega 6 fatty acid consumption and diseases such as cardiovascular disease,

inflammatory conditions such as arthritis, and some types of cancer. In relation to skin health, this can trigger or exacerbate inflammatory lesions such as eczema.

So, it is vital that we get this ratio right. This balancing act can often lead to quite a bit of head scratching and guesswork, so what I recommend is that people focus on getting extra omega 3 into their diet, and don't worry too much about their consumption of omega 6, as generally we tend to get more than enough from the usual array of foods that seem to dominate our diets in this part of the world. This means you should eat plenty of oily fish such as salmon, mackerel, sardines, anchovies and herring.

COMMON SKIN CONDITIONS

ACNE VULGARIS

Acne has got to be one of the most distressing conditions that anyone can suffer from, especially when it is on the face – the only part of our body that is constantly on show. It is a condition that I can relate to very well and is the reason I sit here today writing this book and working in the nutrition world.

Acne has quite a simple cause: too much sebum (oil) is released from the skin's sebaceous glands; or the sebum has an increased viscosity; or there's a combination of the two.

The most widely affected areas for acne are the face and the back, where the highest concentrations of pilosebaceous units are found. Each unit consists of a hair follicle, a hair, a sebaceous gland and the musculature that makes the hair stand up or relax.

The sebaceous glands begin to enlarge and produce higher volumes of sebum when there is an elevation of androgen (i.e. testosterone). A rise in androgen can occur for a whole host of reasons. Most commonly it is as a result of puberty, particularly in young males. However, there are other causes, such as hormonal fluctuations when a woman is using the contraceptive pill, or comes off the pill. It can also occur in cases of polycystic ovary syndrome, where ovarian follicles are not functioning correctly and are releasing higher than normal levels of androgen.

There are several stages in the development of an acne lesion. The first involves small changes within the pilosebaceous unit. An increased production of sebum causes the pore to fill with oil rather rapidly. This then traps dead skin cells that naturally slough off the skin's surface on a daily basis. These cells, along with sebum, and a protein called keratin, can begin to form a plug within the pore, leading to a blockage. This blockage then prevents sebum from exiting the pore and lubricating the skin. This can cause a natural reflex of an increase in sebum production. This initial stage results in a comedone (blackhead).

The next stage is an increase in bacterial numbers within the blocked pore. The bacterium *Propionibacterium acnes* (P. acnes) naturally lives happily within the pore, and ususally isn't prominent enough to create any issues in the local tissue that would lead to infection. The P. acnes bacterium actually uses sebum as a food source. When sebum production increases, it is logical that the number of bacteria will also begin to rise.

As the pore continues to fill with sebum, bacteria and cells, inflammation begins, and the red bump that we associate with the first signs of a spot starts to appear.

The following stage may or may not occur. If sufficient pressure builds up within the pore, then the follicle wall can rupture, causing its contents to leak into the surrounding skin. This will allow the bacteria to cause infection and the immune system starts to intervene. White blood cells begin to rush to the area in order to deal with the infection. As these white blood cells attack the bacteria and destroy them, they themselves die off. The accumulation of these dead white blood cells forms pus, which soon begins to fill the pore. Hence a white head is formed.

TOP ACNE-FIGHTING NUTRIENTS

VITAMIN A

Vitamin A regulates sebaceous secretions and improves skin tone.

VITAMIN C

While vitamin C is often seen as a panacea for virtually every condition, it certainly does have an important role to play in fighting infection and wound-healing. A little extra vitamin C will help active infected acne lesions heal faster, will help in scar-tissue formation, and will also give the immune system support.

ZINC

Zinc regulates the way in which androgen hormones influence the sebaceous glands, reducing excessive sebum production. Zinc is also involved in the coding of genes within key white blood cells that regulate the way in which these cells respond to infection. This will help support the management of the bacterial infection.

OMEGA 3 FATTY ACIDS

These are probably the best nutrients to reduce the appearance of, and speed up the healing time of, active acne lesions. This is because they help the body to manufacture its own intrinsic anti-inflammatory compounds called prostaglandins. These are by-products produced in the body from metabolising dietary fatty acids, and are involved in the management of the inflammatory response. Omega 3 fatty acids enable us to produce the types of prostaglandin that actually reduce inflammation, so can help to reduce the redness and swelling of an active spot.

FAT-SOLUBLE ANTIOXIDANTS

These are vital for helping to manage inflammation in any active skin lesions. This is because a certain degree of the inflammatory response is instigated by a localised free radical release by white blood cells, so additional antioxidants will help to buffer this. The fat-soluble antioxidants are the only ones that can deliver

this activity through dietary consumption alone. These are compounds such as the carotenoids (beta-carotene, alpha-carotene, astaxanthin and so on), which will naturally begin to make their way into the upper layers of the skin where they can deliver their activity.

★ TOP ACNE-FIGHTING FOODS

- Pumpkin seeds – a great source of zinc and omega 3 fatty acids.
- Prawns – a great source of zinc, selenium and the powerful carotenoid astaxanthin.
- Red (bell) peppers – a source of anti-inflammatory beta-carotene and vitamin C.
- Sweet Potatoes – a rich source of beta-carotene and vitamin C.
- Walnuts – a great zinc and omega 3 source.

ECZEMA

Eczema is a condition that plagues millions, and it seems to be getting more common, especially among teens and young adults. It is reasonably common among small children as their bodies develop, but the number of people that go on to develop chronic eczema into early adulthood and beyond is rising at a rate of knots.

Eczema, in essence, is an inflammation of the skin. There are some closely related skin conditions that come under the eczema bracket, such as contact dermatitis, which have been omitted for now, as the primary focus here is atopic eczema. Atopic means that there is a tendency toward acute allergic reactions, which can manifest itself in several ways: eczema, asthma and hay fever. Eczema, asthma and hay fever are, believe it or not, the same condition manifesting in different body tissues. These atopic conditions are what we refer to as a type 2 hypersensitivity reaction. This is when our own immune system has, for whatever reason, become overly sensitised to a specific stimulus.

Every time our body is exposed to this specific stimulus (which could be food, a detergent or a cosmetic, for example), our immune system automatically recognises it as a pathological influence, and instigates a response to it. This causes a localised immunological reaction that can lead to inflammation and redness.

We also often find that individuals with one of the above have family members who suffer from one of the other conditions, or themselves go on to develop one of the others.

As there is an allergic element to this condition, antibodies to the specific stimulus are created. There is also a localised release of histamine by a type of white blood cell called a mast cell. When histamine begins to accumulate locally, this will bring on the intense itching that so many eczema sufferers report.

SYMPTOMS OF ECZEMA

REDNESS

The redness that is experienced in the early stages of an eczema flare-up is active inflammation in action. When the immune system realises that the body has been exposed to the stimulus, it quickly recruits lots of white blood cells, and sends them off to the skin. When these blood cells arrive at the skin, they leach out chemicals that cause the blood vessels to widen. This widening of the blood vessels allows the white blood cells to move into tissues more rapidly, as well as causing the skin to redden. It also allows some of the watery portion of the blood, the plasma, to leach out into surrounding tissue. This causes the swelling that accompanies redness when inflammation is active.

DRY SKIN

Many eczema sufferers experience dry skin. This occurs as a secondary result of the inflammatory events during the early stages of a flare-up. Inflammation can affect circulation to the sebaceous glands, reduce levels of sebum in the skin, and cause water loss from the skin cells. This leads to skin that is dry and shrivelled, and quick to flake off. The inflammation can also affect the skin cells in a multitude of ways and to such a degree that they will stop functioning normally. This means they die off faster than usual, causing a flaky appearance.

ITCHING

One of the most distressing symptoms of eczema is the chronic itching that accompanies a flare-up. The itching is caused by the localized release of histamine by a mast cell. As histamine accumulates in an area, it facilitates many chemical reactions locally, but also stimulates pain receptors in a specific way. When histamine stimulates nociceptors (pain receptors at nerve endings), the sensation experienced is an intense itching, which can drive sufferers to distraction.

TOP ECZEMA-FIGHTING NUTRIENTS

OMEGA 3 FATTY ACIDS

These vital nutrients have several important roles to play in the management of eczema. Firstly, and most superficially, they help the skin to retain more moisture by enhancing the fluidity of skin cell membranes.

The most important application of omega 3 fatty acids, however, is to manage flare-ups. During the first stages of a flare-up, there is a huge amount of active inflammation taking place. The right types of fatty acids can help our body fight inflammation by allowing it to create its own natural anti-inflammatory compounds known as prostaglandins.

Omega 3 fatty acids, such as those found in oily fish and some types of seeds, will increase the production of series 1 and series 3 prostaglandins, which are natural anti-inflammatories.

B VITAMINS

These are among the most important nutrients for the health of the skin, as they support it on so many levels. As a group, they will support the microcirculation to the outer layers of the skin, which helps to ensure adequate delivery of oxygen and nutrients to, and carry away waste products from, skin cells. This activity has the added bonus of improving skin tone and pigmentation.

The B vitamins are also involved in regulating the turnover of skin cells, and can help to reduce flakiness. They help with the proper metabolism and utilisation of essential fatty acids, so a good intake is important when consuming extra fatty acids of any kind.

FAT-SOLUBLE ANTIOXIDANTS

This type of antioxidant, which includes beta-carotene, and certain flavonoids can be of great use in managing any type of inflammatory skin lesion, for the simple fact they deliver localised antioxidant activity. Some aspects of the inflammatory response are instigated by the local release of free radicals from white blood cells. Adding some antioxidants can help to buffer this. However, it is important that we select the right types of antioxidant in order to achieve this. We need to consume antioxidants that are fat-soluble so that they will make their way into the skin (see the antioxidants chapter for more details). The ideal group for this is the carotenoids. These are the compounds that give foods such as carrots, sweet potatoes and mangoes their vivid orange colour.

★ TOP ECZEMA-FIGHTING FOODS

- Oily fish (salmon, mackerel and herring, for example) – packed to the hilt with inflammation-busting omega 3 fatty acids.
- Brown rice – full of B vitamins.
- Sweet potatoes, carrots and mangoes – full of the potent fat-soluble antioxidant beta-carotene.

ERYTHEMA NODOSUM

Erythema nodosum is a painful inflammatory skin disorder that affects the fatty layer of the skin. It presents itself as very tender red, smooth nodules on the shins, trunk, thighs, face and neck. It is a lesion that often is short lived and follows some other type of physiological event – essentially a transient hypersensitivity reaction.

As it is a semi-acute, self-limiting condition, there is nothing from a dietary perspective that can be done to prevent the condition, but there is certainly a lot that can be done from a treatment point of view. Heavy consumption of the right kind of foods can notably increase healing time.

TOP ERYTHEMA NODOSUM-FIGHTING NUTRIENTS

OMEGA 3 FATTY ACIDS

Yes, fatty acids again! I can't emphasise strongly enough how important these nutrients are for managing any kind of inflammatory issue, be it in the skin or anywhere else in the body. A good intake of fatty acids will help erythema nodosum lesions to ease just that little bit faster.

FAT-SOLUBLE ANTIOXIDANTS

These antioxidants, such as beta-carotene, can help with inflammatory issues. However, as they are fat-soluble, and erythema nodosum affects the fatty layer of the skin, their consumption becomes even more relevant. As fat-soluble compounds, these antioxidants will begin to naturally migrate into this fatty layer of the skin. It is here that they may help to buffer some of the inflammatory activity. Some elements of the inflammatory response involve a localised release of free radicals, so extra targeted antioxidants can make a big difference to the severity of the lesion.

★ TOP ERYTHEMA NODOSUM-FIGHTING FOODS

- Sweet potatoes, carrots, mangoes – all rich sources of the fat-soluble antioxidant beta-carotene.
- Oily fish (such as salmon, mackerel, sardines, anchovies) – rich sources of omega 3 fatty acids.
- Nuts and seeds (such as walnuts, flax and hemp seeds) – rich sources of omega 3 fatty acids.

- Whole grains – such as brown rice, quinoa and oats to provide extra B vitamins for optimal skin tissue health.

KERATOSIS PILARIS

Keratosis pilaris is a condition that I see a lot – not only with clients, but also when I'm out and about, and I bet you have too. It displays itself as small, sandpapery reddish-pink bumps, most commonly found on the backs of the arms but it also appears on the thighs and buttocks. Affected areas can turn darker sometimes too. It often can worsen during pregnancy and does have a tendency to improve with age.

Keratosis pilaris has similarities with one of the early stages of acne. This is the blockage of a hair follicle with keratin, a protein in the skin. This blockage then causes pressure to build within the follicle, and the contents bulge out, creating the little bumps.

TOP KERATOSIS PILARIS-FIGHTING NUTRIENTS

VITAMIN A

Vitamin A is the most important nutrient when it comes to managing keratin production. If too much keratin is being produced too quickly, or if not enough is being produced, then additional vitamin A in the diet can help to regulate this. Reducing any excessive keratin production can notably decrease the severity of keratosis pilaris lesions.

B VITAMINS

This group of vitamins are great for virtually every aspect of skin health. They are of particular use in regulating the turnover of skin cells.

Apart from excessive keratin in the hair follicle, the other factor that contributes to the formation of these bumps is blockage with dead skin cells. If we are shedding skin cells too quickly, this may aggravate the process. Extra B vitamins can help to regulate the turnover of cells.

LICHEN PLANUS

Lichen planus is a condition that is inflammatory in origin. It affects the arms, legs, scalp, mouth and mucous membranes of the vagina. Its exact cause still remains something of a mystery, although it is understood that it is not infectious, doesn't run in families, and cannot be passed to others. It is a non-specific inflammatory lesion.

It appears as small, multi-sided bumps that grow together in clumps, and which can develop scaly areas. The one thing unique to lichen planus, which makes it distinctive from other similar lesions such as eczema and psoriasis, is its notorious lilac/violet colour.

TOP LICHEN PLANUS-FIGHTING NUTRIENTS

OMEGA 3 FATTY ACIDS

The firm favourites for tackling any kind of inflammatory condition. They are beneficial because they help the body to create its own natural anti-inflammatory compounds called prostaglandins.

SELENIUM

Some empirical data suggests that increased selenium intake can have beneficial effects upon the severity of lichen planus lesions. This is most likely due to production of antioxidant enzymes that help to reduce the severity of inflammation.

★ TOP FOODS FOR LICHEN PLANUS

- Oily fish (salmon, mackerel, sardines, anchovies, herring), flax seeds, hemp seeds – packed with anti-inflammatory omega 3 fatty acids.
- Brazil nuts – packed with selenium. Just three Brazil nuts a day can give the full Recommended Daily Allowance (RDA) of selenium.

PSORIASIS

Psoriasis is another relatively common skin disorder, affecting in the region of two per cent of the population. There is no pattern with regards to age or sex.

Psoriasis is a condition that affects the rate of turnover of skin cells. As was discussed earlier, new skin cells are formed at the very bottom layer of the skin, and gradually move upwards through the different layers until they reach the upper layer and are sloughed away. The new cells reach the upper layer in around three to four weeks. However, in cases of psoriasis, this whole sequence is moving at light speed and can happen in as little as three to four days.

There is a chain of thought that believes psoriasis arises as a result of a default in the immune system. This theory involves a group of white blood cells called T cells that migrate to the dermis, and release a series of chemical messengers called cytokines that cause localised inflammation, which in turn will cause a more rapid dying off and turnover of skin cells.

The psoriasis lesion appears as haphazard patches of redness, with a silvery-coloured, flaky scaliness in the centre.

TOP PSORIASIS-FIGHTING NUTRIENTS

OMEGA 3 FATTY ACIDS

These beauties come up a lot in this book, and rightly so. They are one of the most profound groups of nutrients for both maintenance of skin health and also the treatment of many common skin conditions. In psoriasis, regardless of whether the immunological theory is correct, there is certainly a degree of inflammation. This can be observed during a flare-up, when the patches of redness are formed. This redness indicates active inflammation. Omega 3 helps the body to create its own natural anti-inflammatory compounds, the prostaglandins, which can aid in the reduction of the redness that accompanies psoriasis. While this doesn't necessarily stop the condition from arising in the first place, it certainly offers some considerable benefit in the management of its symptoms.

The other benefit of increasing omega 3 fatty acid intake is that it will help to keep the skin more moist. One of the symptoms of psoriasis is the dry flakiness of the skin in the centre of the lesions. While the flakiness is caused by accelerated skin cell turnover, its appearance can be reduced by making the skin able to retain moisture better.

QUERCETIN

Quercetin is a powerful flavonoid (flavonoids are a family of phytochemicals) that has commonly been used for conditions such as hay fever and other allergies.

However, new findings suggest that it may have a role to play in the management of inflammatory skin lesions. This is because quercetin inhibits an enzyme in the body called phospholipase. This enzyme is involved in the production of a fatty acid derivative called arachidonic acid.

As mentioned earlier, a group of communication molecules called prostaglandins is involved in regulating the inflammatory response.

Some prostaglandins switch inflammation on, whereas others switch it off. Arachidonic acid is responsible for the formation of the type of prostaglandins that switch on inflammation. Therefore, inhibiting arachidonic acid release from the cell membrane will reduce the presence of proinflammatory prostaglandins and aid in the reduction in appearance of inflammatory skin lesions.

B VITAMINS

Again, this group is another favourite in any skin condition.

The B vitamins become especially important in psoriasis, as one of their roles is the regulation of skin cell turnover. It is believed that adequate B vitamin intake can slow down skin cell turnover in psoriasis patients.

The most important of the B vitamins here is folate, which is directly associated with skin cell turnover, although the other B vitamins offer support too. While the evidence for this remains unclear, what is certain is that adequate B vitamin intake can certainly improve the overall appearance of the lesions, and also improve skin tone overall.

★ TOP PSORIASIS-FIGHTING FOODS

- Garlic – contains a compound that inhibits lipoxygenase, an enzyme involved in arachidonic acid activity.
- Red onions – a rich source of quercetin.
- Oily fish (salmon, mackerel, sardines, anchovies, herring) – great sources of omega 3 fatty acids.

- Whole grains – such as brown rice, quinoa and oats are a rich source of B vitamins.

OTHER REMEDIES OF INTEREST

VITAMIN D CREAMS

These have become more and more popular in both the natural and conventional treatment of psoriasis. Research has found that vitamin D increases the binding of a peptide (communication protein) called cathelicidin to DNA, which causes a notable inhibition of the specific inflammatory response involved in the instigation of psoriasis lesions. Research is in its early days and there is still little clarity as to whether dietary vitamin D will interact with the condition in the same way. But it is food for thought.

ROSACEA

Rosacea is a distressing skin condition that, while not medically serious, can cause a huge amount of personal problems, due to the fact that it affects the face. It is characterized by facial redness, sometimes with the addition of small spots. Some cases also involve permanent dilation of blood vessels in affected areas.

In some very advanced cases, lobules can form on the nose, giving a bumpy, even bulbous, appearance.

There have been several causative factors linked with rosacea. It is likely that each of these influences will create an environment or biological scenario that will allow the condition to develop.

SKIN FLUSHING

One of the major factors believed to instigate rosacea is prolonged flushing of the skin. This can be caused by a variety of factors such as exposure to varying temperatures (going from cold to hot very rapidly), regular heavy exercise and even excessive alcohol consumption. All of these lead to vascular changes and dilation of blood vessels. Usually the blood vessels return to normal in a matter of minutes, but continual fluctuations, and the strain this places upon the musculature of the vessel walls, can lead to permanent dilation.

GUT MICROBIOME

There is now an apparent link between disturbances in gut bacteria composition and rosacea. Recent studies have used the hydrogen breath test, where a positive result indicates the overgrowth of bad bacteria within the small intestine. Patients with rosacea were more often hydrogen positive than those patients in the trial who did not suffer from the condition. When these patients were treated with antibiotics, their rosacea symptoms cleared rapidly.

The exact link between the bacterial overgrowth and the onset of rosacea symptoms is not 100 per cent clear, but certainly highlights an interesting therapeutic approach.

TOP ROSACEA-FIGHTING NUTRIENTS

OMEGA 3 FATTY ACIDS

There will be a certain degree of inflammation present in rosacea, especially if there are any spots or pimples. These essential fatty acids will help the body to create its own natural anti-inflammatory compounds, called prostaglandins, which can help to reduce the severity of these lesions.

B VITAMINS

As with other skin conditions, B vitamins play a vital part in the management of rosacea. This is because they help to maintain the day-to-day functionality of the skin. They regulate everything from microcirculation to the outer layers, to the turnover of skin cells.

PROBIOTIC BACTERIA

These probably represent one of the most exciting natural approaches to treatment of this condition. As discussed above, there is a link between the overgrowth of certain types of bad bacteria in the small intestine and rosacea. While antibiotic treatments have proved successful in the past, it is my belief that such medications should only be used in conditions that are life-threatening, such as sepsis or acute infection, unless there really is no other option. Instead, one of the most powerful, safe and natural ways of dealing with such overgrowths is to ensure that we have a very healthy gut flora, by providing ample amounts of the good bacteria that live in our gut. These good bacteria offer a million and one beneficial effects to our health, from regulating the activity of gut tissue, to acting as a physical barrier to pathogenic organisms, to regulating localised and systemic immune responses.

Good bacteria in the gut are the first line of defence if any other types of bacteria decide to try their luck and cause problems within our digestive tract. They soon wipe the bad bacteria out and make sure they don't go anywhere they are not supposed to. Regular supplementation with probiotic cultures and following a diet that is rich in prebiotic compounds (see below) are recommended.

★ TOP FOODS FOR ROSACEA

- Oily fish (salmon, mackerel, anchovies, sardines, herring) – high in omega 3 fatty acids.
- Red onions – these contain a prebiotic agent, inulin, that encourages the growth of good bacteria.
- Simply cooked dishes – too much spice and seasoning can cause excessive flushing.
- Brightly coloured fruit and vegetables – these bright colour pigments generally represent antioxidant compounds.

FOODS TO AVOID

SPICY FOODS

In some individuals, rosacea is caused or aggravated by facial flushing. Some spicy foods can rapidly cause flushing and, as a result, can worsen the condition.

Chillies, for example, contain a powerful phytochemical called capsaicin – the stuff that actually burns your tongue. This compound can interact with the smooth muscle walls of the blood vessels, and cause them to relax. This leads to a widening of the vessel, which will, in turn, stimulate circulation and flushing.

Ginger is another spice that can have this effect. The essential oils in ginger that give it its spicy flavour will have a similar effect to chillies as they cause relaxation of the blood vessels and the accompanying flushing.

THE RECIPES

BREAKFASTS

SMOKED SALMON, SPINACH AND TOMATO SAVOURY MUFFINS

MAKES 6–8 MUFFINS

6 medium eggs
olive oil, for greasing
100g smoked salmon
2 handfuls of baby spinach,
    wilted
8 cherry tomatoes, quartered
40g feta cheese
sea salt and black pepper

Savoury muffins may sound like some kind of bakery nightmare, but really they are very palatable. I like to use a silicone muffin tray to bake them in, as it is easier to get them out. If you don't have one of these, you can use paper muffin cases.

1. Preheat the oven to 180°C/160°C fan/350°F/gas mark 4.

2. Crack the eggs into a bowl and whisk well.

3. If you're using a muffin tray, grease it with a little oil.

4. Divide the salmon, wilted spinach and tomatoes between each muffin space and pour the whisked eggs into each one.

5. Crumble over the feta, then season with salt and pepper.

6. Bake in the oven for 15–20 minutes. Slide a knife into one of the muffins. If it comes out clean, they are cooked, if there is any liquid egg on the knife, they need a little longer.

BENEFITS

EGGS – A fantastic source of so many nutrients. They are particularly rich in B vitamins, vital for overall skin health.

SALMON – Rich in anti-inflammatory omega 3 fatty acids.

SPINACH – Surprisingly rich in beta-carotene.

AVOCADO, TOMATO, ONION, CHILLI, AND CHEDDAR OMELETTE

SERVES 1

2 large eggs
olive oil, for frying
½ ripe avocado, diced
¼ red onion, finely chopped
3 small tomatoes, chopped
1 small red chilli, finely
  chopped
a handful of grated mature
  cheddar

This is a lovely flavoursome omelette that will keep you full for hours, and provides a big whack of nutrition in your first meal of the day.

1. Crack the eggs into a bowl and whisk.

2. Place a small amount of olive oil in a large heavy-based frying pan, over a high heat.

3. Pour in the eggs and allow them to cook until they begin to firm up.

4. Add the avocado, onion, tomatoes, chilli, and cheddar on one side. With a spatula, ease around the edges of the omelette and fold it in half. Continue to cook for 3–4 minutes until the cheese melts.

BENEFITS

EGGS – Rich in B vitamins that regulate many aspects of overall skin health.

AVOCADO – Rich in the fat-soluble antioxidant vitamin E.

SWEET POTATO ROSTI WITH GUACAMOLE AND POACHED EGGS

MAKES 1 LARGE BREAK-FAST, OR 2 SMALLER

1 large sweet potato, peeled and grated
2 eggs (1 beaten, 1 left for poaching)
1 large ripe avocado
1 large clove of garlic, finely chopped
½ red onion, very finely chopped
1 small red chilli, finely chopped
juice of ½ a lime
olive oil, for frying
sea salt and black pepper

This makes for a perfect weekend breakfast or brunch with loved ones. Depending on the day ahead, you may want to leave out the garlic, but garlic has many useful properties so I'd advise keeping it in.

1. Place the grated sweet potato between some kitchen paper and squeeze out any excess liquid. Then place in a bowl.

2. Add the beaten egg and mix well.

3. Scoop the flesh of the avocado into another bowl. Add the garlic, onion, chilli, and lime juice, along with a pinch of salt and pepper. Mash together to make a guacamole.

4. Form the sweet potato and egg mixture into a rosti and pan fry in a little olive oil for 4–5 minutes on either side until golden brown.

5. Poach the second egg according to your taste.

6. Serve by dolloping a spoonful of guacamole on top of the rosti, then place the poached egg on top.

BENEFITS

SWEET POTATOES – The bright orange flesh of these beauties comes from very high concentrations of beta-carotene.

EGGS – Rich in B vitamins and the carotenoid lycopene.

KIPPER QUINOA KEDGEREE

SERVES 1

½ red onion, finely chopped
olive oil, for frying
1 teaspoon curry powder
60g (dry weight) quinoa
1 kipper fillet
1 hard-boiled egg
sea salt and black pepper

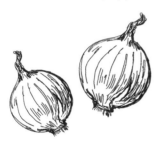

This is a lower-glycaemic and more nutrient-dense variation of the classic rice and fish dish.

1. In a pan, sauté the onion in a little olive oil, along with a pinch of salt, until the onion softens.

2. Add the curry powder and quinoa, and enough water to cover the quinoa. Simmer until the liquid has been absorbed and the quinoa is cooked.

3. While the quinoa is simmering, cook the kipper according to the instructions. If it's not boil-in-the-bag, cook under the grill for 10–15 minutes. Once cooked, flake the fish.

4. Peel and chop the hard-boiled egg. Combine with the fish and cooked quinoa, and season to taste.

BENEFITS

KIPPERS – These often forgotten breakfast classics are packed with omega 3 fatty acids.

QUINOA – A much lower-glycaemic alternative to rice. Remember that high-glycaemic carbohydrates can be to inflammation what petrol is to a bonfire. Lower-glycaemic alternatives prevent blood sugar spikes. Quinoa has the added benefit of being rich in B vitamins.

BRAZIL NUT, WALNUT AND PUMPKIN SEED MUESLI

SERVES 1

4 tablespoons porridge oats
1 tablespoon chopped
  walnuts
1 tablespoon chopped
  Brazil nuts
1 tablespoon pumpkin seeds

This lovely recipe contains a broad spectrum of skin-loving nutrients so you will get your skin-nourishing day off to a flying start.

Nice and easy. Combine all the ingredients in a bowl and serve with rice milk, or other non-dairy milk, or natural live yogurt. You could even scatter a few blueberries over to bump up the nutrient levels . . . not that it needs it!

BENEFITS

OATS – Packed with B vitamins, the nutritional regulators of all aspects of skin health. They are especially rich in biotin, which maintains the health of skin cells but also plays a vital role in the body's ability to correctly utilise fatty acids.

WALNUTS – True superstars. Research on these wonderful nuts has shown that their high oil content is a massive 94 per cent omega 3 fatty acids! This makes them one of the richest sources of these vital fats on the planet. Walnuts are also very high in zinc. Anyone with acne or eczema that has a tendency to become infected should definitely increase their zinc intake as its supportive effect on immune function can reduce the severity of such conditions.

BRAZIL NUTS – Brazils are another nutritional powerhouse. They are one of the richest sources of selenium, the cofactor in the production of glutathione peroxidase – a powerful antioxidant enzyme that is produced naturally within the body. While offering antioxidant protection to all tissues, glutathione peroxidase can also play a role in managing inflammation. This means that any areas of redness that occur during flare-ups may be reduced by increasing selenium intake.

PUMPKIN SEEDS – Another very rich source of zinc and therefore offer nutritional support to the immune system, useful for fighting acne and other infected skin lesions. They are also reasonably high in essential fatty acids. However, there are equal amounts of omega 6 and omega 3 in pumpkin seeds, so don't go too crazy with how many you consume as it is vital that we maintain that all-important ratio of twice the amount of omega 3 to omega 6 each day.

SMOKED SALMON EGGS BENEDICT

SERVES 1

2 eggs
hollandaise sauce
  (OK, I admit it, I tend to buy
  a fresh readymade one, but
  feel free to make your own if
  you want)
½ wholemeal English muffin
2–3 slices of smoked salmon

This is my all-time favourite breakfast! I eat it at least four or five times a week. It is seriously nutrient-dense, tastes amazing, and is really rather a decadent affair too!

1. Crack both eggs gently into a pan of boiling water, and poach for 3–4 minutes.

2. Warm the hollandaise sauce in a small pan.

3. Toast the muffin half and place the smoked salmon slices on top.

4. Place the poached eggs on top of the salmon.

5. Top the whole lot with enough hollandaise sauce to cover it well.

BENEFITS

EGGS – Eggs have got a bad rap over the years, but unjustly so. They are nutritional powerhouses. They are a very rich source of the B vitamins, so can improve the skin's overall functioning as the B vitamins regulate almost all metabolic activity within the different layers of the skin. Provided that the eggs are of reasonable quality, they should also provide a fair amount of omega 3 fatty acids too.

SALMON – A wonderful source of omega 3 fatty acids, the skin's best friends. These vital fats will maintain the moisture and fluidity of skin cells. Salmon is also a rich source of the trace mineral selenium. This nutrient is the cofactor for the antioxidant enzyme glutathione peroxidase, which is able to protect almost every tissue from free radical damage.

BREAKFAST SMOOTHIE

SERVES 1

2 handfuls of frozen mixed
  berries
200ml rice milk or almond
  milk
1 scoop of whey protein
  powder (vanilla works
  best here)
2 tablespoons flaxseed oil

This is a quick and easy morning smoothie that you can run out the door with. Convenience is always good.

Place all the ingredients into a blender, and blend into a thick luscious smoothie.

BENEFITS

BERRIES – All berries will naturally be rich in a range of antioxidant compounds. Having a mixture of different types of berries here will provide a broader scope of antioxidants, as different colour pigments relate to different types of antioxidants. Some of these will come into the fat-soluble category, so will offer those protective benefits to the fatty subcutaneous layer of the skin.

WHEY PROTEIN POWDER – The protein powder has been included here to regulate the impact this smoothie has on blood sugar levels. Fruit contains fast-releasing sugars, which can cause a sharp rise in blood sugar. Continual sharp rises in blood sugar can lead to cross-linking of collagen fibres, causing the skin to lose elasticity, and age prematurely. Adding a scoop of protein powder changes the whole picture. It causes the sugars to enter the blood at a slower rate, and it will have the added bonus of keeping you fuller for longer.

FLAXSEED OIL – A very good source of omega 3 fatty acids. While it doesn't provide the full spectrum of these vital components in the same way that oily fish does, it does come pretty close. So this lovely light-tasting oil should be another addition to your daily routine for plump, smooth skin.

SPINACH AND FETA BREAKFAST SCRAMBLE

SERVES 1

2 handfuls of baby spinach
olive oil, for frying
3 medium eggs
80g feta cheese, cubed

This is a gorgeous dish. Be warned though, it's only for those days when you are extra hungry as it's very filling!

1. Add the baby spinach to a pan with a little olive oil and sauté until it wilts.

2. Crack the eggs into a bowl, and whisk them with a fork.

3. Add the eggs to the pan with the spinach and stir continuously over a high heat. As soon as the eggs start to scramble, add in the feta and continue stirring.

4. Once all the egg is scrambled, it is ready to serve.

BENEFITS

EGGS – Packed with B vitamins to support daily skin function, and also the essential fatty acids.

SPINACH – Packed with a ridiculous amount of goodies. It is a very rich source of beta-carotene, one of the most powerful fat-soluble antioxidants and therefore able to offer its support in the subcutaneous layer of the skin.

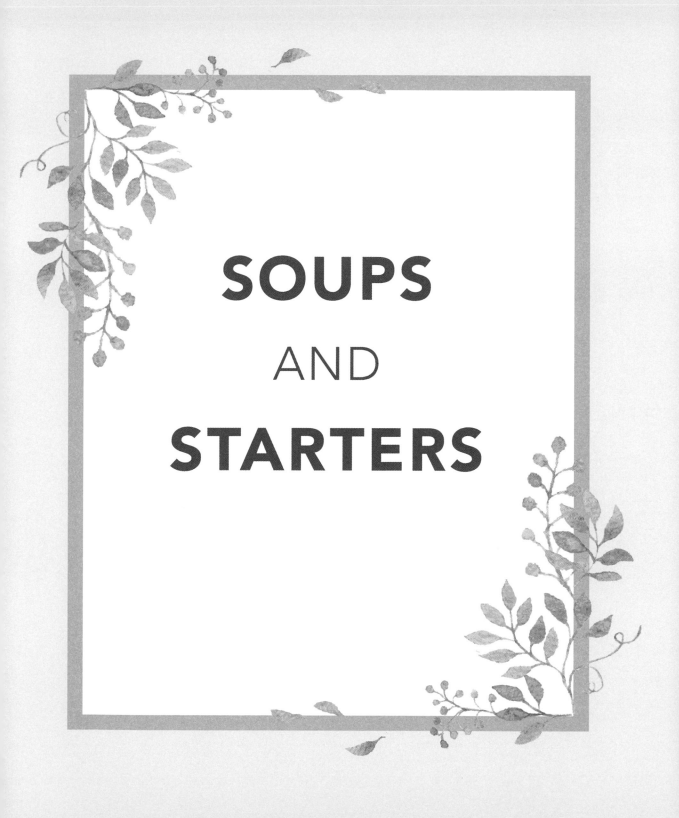

SOUPS
AND
STARTERS

BEETROOT AND HORSERADISH SOUP

SERVES 1–2

1 red onion, finely sliced
olive oil, for frying
1 large potato, diced
1 bunch of medium beetroot, washed and diced
vegetable stock
3 tablespoons horseradish sauce
sea salt

This bright-purple powerhouse will get you tingling all over.

1. In a saucepan, sauté the onion in a little olive oil, along with a generous pinch of salt, until the onion has softened.

2. Add the potato and beetroot, cover with enough stock to just cover the ingredients and simmer until the vegetables soften.

3. Add the horseradish sauce, then use a hand blender or add to a food processor and blend to make a thick velvety soup.

BENEFITS

BEETROOT – Contains some very interesting and powerful chemistry. There is a group of phytochemicals called betalains, one of which, betacyanin, is responsible for the deep purple colour of beetroot. Betalains have been shown to influence liver function by ramping up the glutathione enzymatic system, which is part of the series of processes that break down and remove waste products from the body. Beetroot is also very rich in the powerful antioxidant compound zeaxanthin, which protects the fatty subcutaneous tissue from damage. Free radical-mediated damage to this tissue can have significant impact upon the skin becoming saggy and dull.

TOMATO AND FENNEL SOUP

SERVES 2–4

2 tablespoons olive oil
1 large red onion, finely
 chopped
2 cloves of garlic, finely
 chopped
1 small fennel bulb, finely
 chopped
1 teaspoon crushed fennel
 seeds
2 x 400g tins of chopped
 tomatoes
3 tablespoons orange juice
vegetable stock
sea salt

I have to admit, I don't make my own vegetable stock but just use a good quality vegetable bouillon. I generally make up a litre and add however much is needed to the recipe, storing any leftover in the fridge for the next day, or in the freezer for later use.

1. Add the olive oil, chopped onion, chopped garlic and chopped fennel, along with a generous pinch of salt, to a saucepan, and sauté until the onion and fennel have softened.

2. Add the fennel seeds, tomatoes and orange juice. Then add enough stock to just cover the ingredients.

3. Simmer for 10 minutes.

4. Use a hand blender to blend into a smooth, vibrant soup. Season to taste.

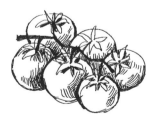

BENEFITS

ONIONS AND GARLIC – Like all members of the allium family, they are very rich in sulphur. Sulphur is a key component of the extracellular matrix, the lattice-like network of fibres that gives the skin structural support.

FENNEL – A great source of B vitamins, vital for overall skin health. Fennel is also rich in fibre for improved digestion.

TOMATOES – Are bursting with some powerful antioxidant compounds. They are high in beta-carotene and lycopene, another carotenoid compound. Both of these are fat-soluble antioxidants.

PROPER BELL PEPPER SOUP

SERVES 2–4

1 red onion, coarsely
   chopped
2 cloves of garlic, finely
   chopped
olive, oil for frying
3 red bell peppers, coarsely
   chopped
1 large sweet potato, diced
vegetable stock
sea salt

This soup is gorgeous and nutrient-rich. Serve with a nice hunk of fresh wholemeal bread, and get transported to heaven!

1. In a saucepan, sauté the onion and garlic in a little olive oil, along with a pinch of salt, until the onion has softened.

2. Add the peppers and sweet potato and enough vegetable stock to just cover the ingredients, and simmer until the potatoes have softened.

3. Use a hand blender, or add to a food processor, and blend into a smooth soup.

BENEFITS

RED BELL PEPPERS – Bursting with a whole range of powerful compounds. The phytochemicals responsible for the vivid red colour are called flavonoids, which have very powerful antioxidant properties. All varieties of bell pepper contain a large amount of beta-carotene, another colour pigment ranging from yellow to deep orange. Beta-carotene is a fat-soluble antioxidant, which means it will be most active within fatty tissues, especially the fatty subcutaneous layer of the skin. This will help to protect the skin from free radical damage, and can help to maintain elasticity and plumpness.

Helpful hint: When buying red bell peppers, buy ones with the deepest colour that you can find. The darker they are, the higher the concentration of the anti-oxidant flavonoids.

SWEET POTATOES – Very rich sources of beta-carotene. It is this compound that is responsible for the vivid orange colour of their flesh.

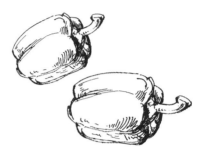

SPICED PARSNIP SOUP

SERVES 2–4

1 large white onion, coarsely
  chopped
1 clove of garlic, finely
  chopped
2.5cm piece of ginger, peeled
  and finely chopped
½ teaspoon cinnamon
½ teaspoon mild curry
  powder
olive oil, for frying
6 parsnips, cut into chunks
vegetable stock
sea salt

This delectable soup is a digestive dynamo. The better your digestion, the better your skin!

1. In a saucepan, sauté the onion and garlic, along with the spices and a pinch of salt, in a little olive oil, until the onion softens.

2. Add the chopped parsnips and enough stock to just cover the ingredients. Simmer until the parsnips are soft.

3. Use a hand blender, or add to a food processor, and blend into a smooth soup.

BENEFITS

PARSNIPS – Very rich in a special kind of carbohydrate called fructo-oligosaccharide (FOS), which is a potent prebiotic. Prebiotics stimulate the growth of good bacteria in the digestive tract. These good bacteria help to regulate almost every aspect of digestion and absorption. This has a knock-on effect on many aspects of our health.

ONIONS AND GARLIC – Great sources of the mineral silica, one of the key nutrients for healthy skin.

SPICY BLACK BEAN AND JERUSALEM ARTICHOKE SOUP

SERVES 2–4

1 red onion, finely chopped
2 cloves of garlic, finely
  chopped
1 stick of celery, finely
  chopped
olive oil, for frying
3 Jerusalem artichokes, diced
1 x 400g tin of black beans,
  drained
vegetable stock

This is quite a filling soup, and a great digestive tonic to boot!

1. Add the onion, garlic and celery to a saucepan with a little olive oil, and sauté until the onion softens.

2. Add the Jerusalem artichokes and the black beans, and enough vegetable stock to just cover the ingredients.

3. Simmer until the Jerusalem artichokes soften.

4. Use a hand blender, or add to a food processor, and blend until smooth.

BENEFITS

BLACK BEANS – A rich source of the B vitamins, which help to support almost every aspect of skin health. They are also rich in zinc, which helps regulate oil production in the skin and supports immunity, which can help in managing infected skin lesions.

JERUSALEM ARTICHOKES – Wonderful and unusual vegetables that are another digestive dynamo. They contain special carbohydrates called fructo-oligosaccharides and inulin that work as a food source for the good bacteria in the gut. When gut flora feed on these vital sugars, they start to reproduce, further enhancing the strength of the good gut flora. This will then improve elimination and nutrient absorption.

ROASTED BUTTERNUT SQUASH SOUP

SERVES 3–4

1 large butternut squash, skin
  on, diced
olive oil
1 large red onion, finely
  chopped
3 cloves of garlic, finely
  chopped
500ml vegetable stock (you
  may not need all of this)

This simple yet flavoursome soup is a great beta-carotene hit.

1. Preheat the oven to 180°C/160°C fan/350°F/gas mark 4.

2. Place the cubed butternut squash on a baking tray. Drizzle over a small amount of olive oil and roast in the oven for around 20–25 minutes, stirring occasionally, until the edges are golden and turning crispy.

3. In a saucepan, sauté the onion and garlic in a little olive oil until the onion has softened.

4. Add the roasted squash to the onion and garlic and add enough vegetable stock to just cover the ingredients.

5. Use a hand blender to purée into a smooth soup.

BENEFITS

SQUASH – A high concentration of beta-carotene gives the flesh its orange colour.

CARROT AND CARAWAY SOUP

SERVES 3–4

1 large red onion, finely
   chopped
1 clove of garlic, finely
   chopped
1 tablespoon caraway seeds
olive oil, for frying
5–6 large carrots, chopped
500ml of vegetable stock (you
   may not need all of this)

This is a delicately flavoured, summery soup with fat-soluble antioxidants in abundance.

1. In a saucepan, sauté the onion, garlic, and caraway seeds in a little olive oil until the onion has softened and the seeds are releasing their fragrant oils.

2. Add the chopped carrots and enough vegetable stock to almost cover the ingredients. Simmer until the carrots soften.

3. Use a hand blender, or add to a food processor, and blend into a smooth soup.

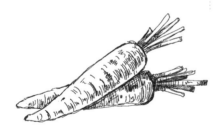

BENEFITS

CARROTS – Very rich in the fat-soluble antioxidant beta-carotene. This compound can accumulate in the fatty subcutaneous layer of the skin where it can offer localised protection against free radicals.

SOUTH–EAST ASIAN SEAFOOD SOUP

SERVES 2–3

1 large red onion, finely
  chopped
3 cloves of garlic, finely
  chopped
1 small red chilli, finely
  chopped
2 stalks of lemongrass, bashed
2 star anise
olive oil, for frying
1 x 400ml tin coconut milk
300ml of vegetable stock (you
  may not need it all)
1 skinless salmon fillet, diced
100g king prawns
juice of 1 lime
1 tablespoon fish sauce
sea salt

This is a beautiful, fragrant, spicy soup that has a broad spectrum of skin-friendly nutrients.

1. In a saucepan, sauté the onion, garlic, chilli, lemongrass and star anise in a little olive oil, along with a pinch of salt, until the onion has softened and the lemongrass and star anise have become fragrant.

2. Add the coconut milk and about 100ml of vegetable stock. Then add the diced salmon and the prawns and simmer until both are cooked.

3. Squeeze in the lime juice and add the fish sauce and stir. If the soup is a bit thick, then thin it out with some more vegetable stock.

4. Remove the lemongrass stalks before serving.

BENEFITS

PRAWNS – A great source of the mineral zinc, which is vital for regulating sebum production. It also supports the immune system in fighting infection.

SALMON – For those all-important omega 3 fatty acids and their potent anti-inflammatory activity.

ROASTED BEETROOT WITH HORSERADISH AND ROCKET SALAD

SERVES 2–4

3 small raw beetroot
olive oil, for drizzling
1 tablespoon horseradish
  sauce
a large handful of fresh rocket
sea salt

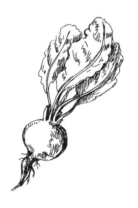

Beetroot are packed with so many skin-healthy nutrients. The marriage of beetroot and horseradish is a match made in heaven.

1. Preheat the oven to 220°C/200°C fan/425°F/gas mark 7.

2. Scrub the beetroot but leave the skins on. Cut into cubes and place in a roasting tin. Drizzle with olive oil and add a generous pinch of salt. Roast in the oven until the beetroot is soft and the skin has become crispy.

3. Place the roasted beetroot in a bowl and stir through a generous dollop of horseradish sauce.

4. Serve over a bed of fresh rocket.

BENEFITS

BEETROOT – A rich source of betalains that have been shown to positively affect liver function.

CROSTINI WITH OLIVE AND ARTICHOKE PÂTÉ

SERVES 2–4

1 x 200g jar of artichoke
  hearts
4 tablespoons chopped
  green olives
3 tablespoons olive oil
good-quality ciabatta bread,
  sliced

This is a flavour explosion and fabulous for the health of the skin.

1. Simply add the artichokes, olives and olive oil to a food processor and blend into a smooth pâté.

2. Spread this luscious pâté on slices of toasted ciabatta, and enjoy as crostini.

BENEFITS

OLIVES – Have long been associated with beauty and skin health. They are a very rich source of the antioxidant nutrient vitamin E. Vitamin E helps to reduce free radical damage within fatty tissues and cell membranes, so it's a vital nutrient for reducing skin ageing and improving overall skin appearance.

SMOKED SALMON WITH ASPARAGUS AND CHILLI LIME DRESSING

SERVES 1

5–6 asparagus spears
3 slices of good-quality
  smoked salmon

for the dressing
juice of ½ a lime
½ red chilli, deseeded and
  finely chopped
1 teaspoon honey
1 tablespoon soy sauce
2 teaspoons toasted
  sesame oil

This very simple salad is light but packed with skin-saving nutrients.

1. In a small container, combine all of the dressing ingredients. Mix well and leave aside.

2. Immerse the asparagus into a pan of boiling water for no longer than 2 minutes, just long enough for it to turn bright green and soften slightly.

3. Lay out the asparagus on a serving plate, and cover with the slices of smoked salmon. Drizzle over the dressing and serve.

BENEFITS

SALMON – A dense source of the all-important omega 3 fatty acids. These fatty acids in the form of EPA and DHA, which are found in all oily fish, can be metabolised to form anti-inflammatory substances called prostaglandins. With many skin issues, such as acne and eczema, there is active inflammation that causes the angry redness. Reducing the inflammation will calm the redness down.

ROASTED SQUASH, WALNUT, FENNEL AND ORANGE SALAD

SERVES 1

½ small butternut squash, skin on, diced
1 small fennel bulb, thinly sliced
2 tablespoons fresh flat leaf parsley, roughly chopped
2 tablespoons walnuts

for the dressing
3 tablespoons orange juice
2 tablespoons extra virgin olive oil
1 clove of garlic, very finely chopped
a pinch of salt
a pinch of black pepper

This is a gorgeous summery salad, bursting with flavour.

1. Preheat the oven to 180°C/ 160°C fan/ 350°F/gas mark 4.

2. Place the diced squash on a baking tray and roast for 20–25 minutes, or until soft with golden edges and crispy skin. Remove and set aside to cool slightly.

3. Mix the dressing ingredients together.

4. Combine the roasted squash, sliced fennel, parsley and walnuts together and toss. Add the dressing, and toss again.

BENEFITS

BUTTERNUT SQUASH – Packed with the fat-soluble antioxidant beta-carotene, which can accumulate in the fatty subcutaneous layer of the skin.

ORANGE – Rich in vitamin C, which is vital for the formation of collagen, the protein that helps to maintain the structural integrity of the skin.

TUNA, MANGO, ROCKET AND RED ONION SALAD

SERVES 1

1 small red onion, peeled and
    cut into wedges
olive oil, for drizzling
½ ripe mango
1 large tuna steak
a large handful of fresh rocket

This is a great combination of ingredients and such an easy lunch to make ahead of your work day and take in as a packed lunch. It's also nutrient-dense, flavoursome and vibrant.

1. Preheat the oven to 180°C/160°C fan/350°F/gas mark 4.

2. Place the onion wedges on to a baking tray, drizzle with olive oil, and roast for 20 minutes, or until soft with the edges beginning to turn crispy.

3. Peel and dice the mango.

4. Pan-fry the tuna steak according to preference.

5. Assemble the salad by tossing together the rocket, mango and roasted onion. Place the tuna steak on top.

BENEFITS

TUNA – Rich in omega 3 fatty acids, but it is the level of minerals and trace minerals it contains that makes it a real hero ingredient. Tuna is rich in both zinc and selenium. Zinc is vital for regulating sebum production and also supporting white blood cell response to infection. Selenium is the cofactor for the major anti-oxidant enzyme glutathione peroxidase.

MANGO – A delightful source of beta-carotene – just look at the orange colour of its sweet flesh.

RAW KALE SALAD WITH AVOCADO, SUN-DRIED TOMATOES, OLIVES AND PARMESAN

SERVES 1

3 handfuls of curly kale
olive oil, for drizzling
½ very ripe avocado
2 tablespoons chopped sun-dried tomatoes
2 tablespoons chopped black olives
3 tablespoons of grated Parmesan
sea salt

This gorgeous salad may sound a little weird at first, but give it a try. You'll find massaging kale is also oddly satisfying! It has plenty of flavour and is nutritionally very dense indeed.

1. Place the kale in a bowl and pick out any thicker, woodier stems. Drizzle over a small amount of olive oil, along with a good pinch of salt, and massage the kale with your hands until the kale softens and wilts.

2. Add the flesh of the avocado to the kale and continue to massage so that the avocado gives the kale a creamy coating.

3. Add the sun-dried tomatoes, olives and Parmesan, and mix well.

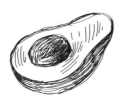

BENEFITS

KALE – A rich source of beta-carotene, the wonderful fat-soluble antioxidant.

PARMESAN – Will help with the absorption of the beta-carotene. As it's a fat-soluble nutrient, having it with something fatty enhances its absorption.

AVOCADO – These weird and wonderful fruits are very rich in the fat-soluble antioxidant vitamin E, which helps to support the health of cell membranes.

ROASTED CARROT AND RED ONION SALAD WITH SALSA VERDE

SERVES 2

4–5 large carrots, cut into
   batons
1 large red onion, cut into
   wedges
olive oil, for drizzling
a handful of baby spinach,
   shredded
1–2 tablespoons crumbled
   goat's cheese

for the salsa verde
1 teaspoon capers
1 teaspoon fresh mint,
   chopped
1 teaspoon fresh basil,
   chopped
1 teaspoon fresh flat leaf
   parsley, chopped
½ teaspoon dijon mustard
½ teaspoon white wine
   vinegar
3 teaspoons extra virgin
   olive oil

This is a great salad that can be served warm in winter, or cold as a summer side dish.

1. Preheat the oven to 180°C/160°C fan/350°F/gas mark 4.

2. Place the carrots and onions on a baking tray, drizzle with olive oil, and roast for 25–30 minutes, or until both are soft and starting to turn golden at the edges.

3. Put the carrots, onions, shredded spinach and crumbled goat's cheese into a bowl and toss together.

4. Mix all of the salsa verde ingredients together, dress the salad with it, and toss well.

BENEFITS

CARROTS – One of the best sources of beta-carotene.

MAIN COURSES

SQUID WITH GARLIC, CHILLI AND LEMONGRASS

SERVES 2

½ red onion, sliced

4 cloves of garlic, finely chopped

1 large red chilli, finely chopped

3 large spring onions, halved then cut into strips

1 large carrot, cut into batons

2 stalks of lemongrass, bashed then halved

150g squid, cut into rings

2 teaspoons honey

2 teaspoons sesame oil

This is a lovely fragrant dish that works great with brown rice, noodles, or stir-fried vegetables.

1. In a pan, sauté the onion, garlic, chilli, spring onions, carrot and lemongrass, until the onion and carrot are beginning to soften.

2. Add the squid and continue to cook for 3–5 minutes, until it is cooked through.

3. Add the honey and sesame oil and stir through before serving.

BENEFITS

SQUID – One of the best sources of zinc around. This mineral is a powerhouse for anyone with acne. It helps reduce over-production of sebum and most importantly is used by white blood cells to code genes that regulate the way in which they fight infection.

COCONUT-CRUSTED SALMON ON SPICED SWEET POTATO PURÉE WITH GARLIC GREENS

SERVES 2

3 tablespoons coconut flour
3 tablespoons desiccated
    coconut
¼ teaspoon garlic powder
a pinch of sea salt
2 salmon fillets
1 egg, whisked
3 handfuls of shredded
    greens (spring greens or
    cavolo nero)
3 cloves of garlic, finely
    chopped

for the purée
½ red onion, finely chopped
olive oil, for frying
1 large sweet potato, peeled
    and diced
1 teaspoon cinnamon
½ teaspoon cumin

Make this for a cosy night in. It's also a gorgeous dish to whip up at a dinner party, if you up the quantities accordingly. There's a bit of a tropical vibe going on here.

1. Preheat the oven to 180°C/160°C fan/350°F/gas mark 4.

2. Mix the coconut flour and desiccated coconut together, along with the garlic powder and salt. Mix well.

3. One at a time dip the salmon fillets into the whisked egg, then roll in the coconut mixture to fully coat.

4. Place the salmon on a baking sheet and bake for around 20 minutes, until the coconut crust turns golden brown.

5. Meanwhile make the purée. Gently fry the chopped onion in the oil until translucent, then add the sweet potato and spices and mix together. Put a lid on the pan and cook over a low heat for around 15 minutes, stirring every now and then to prevent from catching, until the sweet potato is soft.

6. Sauté the greens and garlic together until the greens have wilted.

7. Transfer the spiced sweet potato mix into the bowl of a food processor and blitz until smooth.

8. Place a spoonful of the purée in the centre of each plate. Place a salmon fillet on top of the purée and serve with the wilted greens.

BENEFITS

SALMON – Rich in omega 3 fatty acids.

SWEET POTATO – One of my favourite ways to top up on fat-soluble beta-carotene.

KING PRAWNS IN SATAY SAUCE WITH COCONUT RICE

SERVES 2

1 large red onion, finely sliced
2 cloves of garlic, finely
  chopped
1 red chilli, finely chopped
olive oil, for frying
180g cooked king prawns
1 heaped tablespoon smooth
  peanut butter
2 teaspoons soy sauce
1 teaspoon honey
½ teaspoon Chinese five-
  spice powder
a handful of fresh coriander,
  chopped
sea salt

for the rice
160g brown rice
1 x 400ml tin of coconut milk
2 tablespoons desiccated
  coconut

This is a combination I will never grow tired of. Having spent a great deal of time in Asia, this dish epitomises all the flavours that I love.

1. Place the rice and coconut milk together in a pan and simmer until the coconut milk is absorbed. If the rice is not cooked at this stage, add some water and continue until the rice is fully cooked. Add the desiccated coconut and set aside.

2. In a pan, sauté the onion, garlic and chilli in a little olive oil, along with a pinch of salt, until the onion has softened.

3. Add the prawns and continue to sauté until cooked.

4. Add the peanut butter, soy sauce, honey, five-spice and coriander.

5. Serve the prawns alongside the coconut rice.

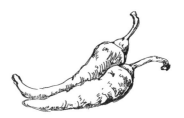

BENEFITS

PRAWNS – Rich in the mineral zinc. Zinc helps to regulate sebum production and speed up the healing of infection.

PEANUT BUTTER – A good source of B vitamins, important for overall skin health.

BROWN RICE – Rich in a variety of B vitamins.

SALMON AND TOMATO SKEWERS WITH NUTTY QUINOA AND SPINACH SALAD

SERVES 1

1 large clove of garlic
a handful of fresh basil leaves
1 tablespoon olive oil
1 large salmon fillet, cut into large cubes
3 cherry tomatoes
40g (dry weight) quinoa
2 teaspoons vegetable stock powder
2 handfuls of baby spinach

This is one of my favourite combinations of ingredients, not only because of the flavours, but also for the way that I feel afte eating it. It always leaves me feeling fantastic and energised.

1. Finely chop the garlic and basil together at the same time, working the two ingredients together to form a coarse paste. Place in a bowl, along with the olive oil, and mix thoroughly to create a marinade. Add in the cubed salmon and mix everything together, ensuring the salmon is well coated in the marinade.

2. Leave in the fridge to marinate for an hour.

3. Remove the salmon from the fridge. Load a skewer with the salmon and the tomatoes alternately.

4. Place the quinoa grains into a suacepan, cover with hot water and the vegetable stock powder and bring to the boil. Turn down the heat and simmer for 20 minutes. When the quinoa has been simmering fo 5 minutes, place the salmon skewers under a hot grill for 15 minutes, turning frequently.

5. Serve the salmon skewer over the cooked quinoa. Add the spinach and tomato side salad, tossed with your favourite dressing.

BENEFITS

SALMON – One of the key players here. It's all about those anti-inflammatory omega 3 fatty acids.

QUINOA – A very nutrient-dense grain. It's protein-rich and contains a number of B vitamins.

MOROCCAN-STYLE VEGGIE TAGINE

SERVES 2–4

2 cloves of garlic, finely
  chopped
1 large red onion, finely
  chopped
coconut oil, for frying
1 medium courgette, sliced
a large handful of dates,
  pitted
1 x 400g tin of chopped
  tomatoes
200g cooked chickpeas
1½ teaspoons cinnamon
sea salt

Rich, spicy and flavoursome, this comforting dish gives you a B vitamin hit, with buckets of flavour to boot.

1. In a saucepan, sauté the garlic and onion in a little coconut oil, with a pinch of salt, until the onion has softened.

2. Add the courgette and dates, and continue to sauté until the courgette begins to soften.

3. Add the chopped tomatoes, chickpeas and cinnamon. Simmer until the sauce becomes a fragrant, sweet, thick delight.

4. Serve with couscous or quinoa, and a good side salad.

BENEFITS

ONIONS AND GARLIC – Like all the alliums, these are rich in organic sulphur. This essential mineral is vital for skin health. It is a key constituent in the protein matrix that supports the skin's structural integrity.

CHICKPEAS – A good source of the mineral zinc, as well as B vitamins.

STEAMED SALMON WITH YOGURT SAUCE ON WILTED GREENS

SERVES 1

1 salmon fillet
a handful of shredded spring
   greens (collard greens)

for the sauce
1 clove of garlic, finely
   chopped
2 spring onions, finely
   chopped
olive oil, for frying
1 small pot of fat-free yogurt
a handful of fresh dill, finely
   chopped

This recipe is divine and incredibly nutrient-dense, yet it's an ideal choice for those evenings when you fancy something light.

1. Place the salmon in a steamer tray, and steam for 15–20 minutes. Salmon is a fast-cooking fish so this should be more than enough.

2. Add the spring greens to the steamer after the salmon has been steaming for 10–12 minutes. Remove them at the same time as you remove the salmon.

3. Prepare the sauce last, just before the dish is ready to serve. In a pan, sauté the garlic and the spring onions in a little olive oil, until they both soften slightly.

4. Transfer the yogurt to a small bowl. Add the garlic and spring onions to the yogurt. Add the chopped dill and mix well.

5. Place the greens in the centre of the plate, then place the salmon on top of them. Spoon the yogurt sauce over the salmon, ready to serve.

BENEFITS

SALMON – Rich in anti-inflammatory omega 3 fatty acids.

GREENS – Most greens are very good sources of beta-carotene. It is usually hidden by the chlorophyll that makes them green. This is why leaves change colour in the autumn. The chlorophyll breaks down to reveal the carotenoids that give the yellow, orange and red colours.

SWEET POTATO AND SPINACH CURRY

SERVES 2–4

2 cloves of garlic, finely
  chopped
1 red onion, finely chopped
coconut oil, for frying
2 tablespoons madras or balti
  curry paste
1 x 400ml tin of coconut milk
2 medium sweet potatoes,
  diced
2 handfuls of baby spinach

This is a quick and easy curry – ideal for a fast, healthy, nutrient-packed meal after a busy day.

1. In a saucepan, sauté the garlic and onion in a little coconut oil until the onion has softened. Stir in the curry paste and sauté for a further 2 minutes.

2. Add the coconut milk and the sweet potatoes and cook until the potatoes are just tender. This should take about 10 minutes.

3. Stir through the spinach until wilted.

4. Serve with brown rice or quinoa.

BENEFITS

SWEET POTATOES – A very rich source of that skin-loving antioxidant beta-carotene. This compound accumulates in the subcutaneous layer of the skin, where it can deliver antioxidant support to the collagen and elastin matrix. Beta-carotene can also deliver some anti-inflammatory activity, which can be useful in angry red skin conditions.

SPINACH – Also a dense source of beta-carotene and other compounds in the carotenoid family.

FANTASTIC FISH PIE

SERVES 2–3

1 large red onion, finely
  chopped
3 cloves of garlic, finely
  chopped
olive oil, for frying
1 x 390g packet of fish pie mix
2 tablespoons full-fat soft
  cheese
1 teaspoon wholegrain
  mustard
10g fresh dill, chopped
150ml vegetable stock
1 large sweet potato, peeled
  and diced
sea salt and black pepper

I do love a fish pie and this version is a powerhouse of skin-friendly nutrients.

1. In a pan, sauté the onion and garlic in a little olive oil, with a pinch of salt, until the onion has softened.

2. Add the fish pie mix, the soft cheese, mustard, dill and vegetable stock. Allow this to simmer for 7–8 minutes until the fish has cooked.

3. Meanwhile, boil the diced sweet potato until soft, then mash with a little salt and pepper until smooth. Heat the oven to 180°C/ 160°C fan/350°F/gas mark 4.

4. Place the cooked fish and sauce in a baking dish. Top with the sweet potato mash, then bake for 15–20 minutes, or until the mash starts to turn slightly golden.

BENEFITS

SWEET POTATO – A rich source of fat-soluble beta-carotene.

SOFT CHEESE – A great replacement here for the usual refined white flour and the fats in the cheese help to enhance the absorption of the beta-carotene.

SALMON – It's all about the anti-inflammatory omega 3.

SESAME SOY TUNA STEAKS WITH SWEET POTATO WEDGES

SERVES 1

2 tablespoons soy sauce
1 tablespoon sesame oil
1 teaspoon honey
1 fresh tuna steak
1 large sweet potato
olive oil, for drizzling

This is seriously filling, but won't overload you with calories – and it contains so much skin-friendly nutrition.

1. Combine the soy sauce, sesame oil and honey together in a bowl. Ensure that all three ingredients are well mixed into a glossy emulsion.

2. Add the tuna steak to the bowl, and keep turning it over until it's thoroughly coated in the marinade. Marinate the steak for an hour, 30 minutes on each side.

3. Once the steak has been marinating for an hour, pre-heat the oven to 220°C/200°C fan/425°F/gas mark 7.

4. Cut the sweet potato into wedges (leaving the skin on), and place in a roasting tin. Drizzle over a little olive oil, toss well, and then roast for 20–25 minutes, stirring occasionally.

BENEFITS

TUNA – A rich source of that ever-wonderful nutrient, omega 3. See page 94 for full details of its virtues.

SWEET POTATO – A rich source of the fat-soluble antioxidant beta-carotene.

THAI PRAWN CURRY

SERVES 2–4

1 red onion, finely chopped

1 clove of garlic, finely
   chopped

1 teaspoon freshly grated
   ginger

coconut oil, for frying

2 tablespoons Thai red curry
   paste

1 x 400g tin of chopped
   tomatoes

1 x 50g sachet of coconut
   cream

400g prawns

a handful of spinach (optional)

I love a good curry, and I am very fond of prawns so this is a winner for me. It's a slight diversion from a true Thai taste because it includes tomatoes, but with the red curry paste and the coconut, it has a wonderful fusion of flavours that is halfway between Indian and Thai. Good stuff!

1. In a pan, sauté the onion, garlic and ginger in a little coconut oil, until the onion softens.

2. Stir in the red curry paste and sauté for a further 2 minutes, until fragrant.

3. Add in the tomatoes and the coconut cream, and simmer for about 8 minutes. This will thicken the sauce considerably.

4. Add in the prawns. If they are cooked, simmer for 3 minutes. If they are raw, simmer for about 8 minutes.

5. At the last minute I sometimes stir in a handful of spinach to add a dash of colour and some extra nutrients.

6. Serve with quinoa and salad.

BENEFITS

PRAWNS – Very dense source of the minerals selenium and zinc. Selenium is commonly deficient in the Western diet yet it's vitally important for the long-term health and protection of all tissues, including the skin. This is because it is the cofactor for the body's important antioxidant enzyme glutathione peroxidase. This is a very powerful antioxidant that can protect tissues from free radical damage.

Zinc regulates the activity of the sebaceous glands, helping to normalize their secretions. It's also vital for regulating the activity of white blood cells, due to its role in controlling genetic activity within these cells. This makes zinc extra important in issues such as acne.

TOMATOES – Rich in another of the fat-soluble antioxidants: lycopene. This antioxidant has long been promoted for male health, but is in fact fabulous for the long-term health of the skin too. As a fat-soluble compound, it will naturally migrate into the fatty subcutaneous layer of the skin, where it can offer protection against free radical damage.

RED ONIONS – One of my favourite ingredients. When it comes to skin health, they have some great things to offer. They are a very rich source of sulphur. This often forgotten mineral is a vital component in the manufacture of all connective tissues, including the extracellular matrix. This is the criss-cross lattice of fibres that helps to give tissues their structure. We need to ensure we have a regular supply of dietary sulphur to maintain it.

SPINACH AND CANNELLINI BEAN CRUMBLE

SERVES 2–4

2 cloves of garlic, finely
   chopped
olive oil, for frying
1 x 400g tin of cooked
   cannellini beans
3 large handfuls of baby
   spinach
5 slices of wholemeal bread
1 tablespoon butter
sea salt

This beautiful, filling dish is proper comfort food. Its title gives no hint of the magical flavours that are created when these ingredients are combined together.

1. In a pan, add the chopped garlic to some very hot oil. This is one of those rare occasions where you want the garlic to actually begin to brown. This gives it a toasted flavour.

2. Half drain the cannellini beans, and add them to the garlic, along with the remaining liquid from the tin and a pinch of salt. Simmer for a minute, before adding the spinach.

3. Place the bread in a food processor and blitz to make breadcrumbs.

4. Melt the butter in a pan. Once melted, add the breadcrumbs to the butter and mix thoroughly.

5. Preheat the oven to 200°C/180°C fan/400°F/gas mark 6.

6. Place the cannellini bean mixture in a baking dish and top with the buttered breadcrumbs. Bake in the oven until the topping has turned golden brown.

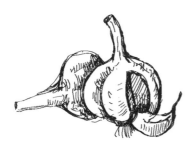

BENEFITS

CANNELLINI BEANS – One of the frequently neglected parts of the skin health picture is good digestion and proper elimination of waste products. If we are not eliminating properly through regular bowel movements (and believe me, it's quite an epidemic these days), we start to create a rather nasty environment within our digestive tract. Waste products that don't leave the gut quickly enough can start to be absorbed back through the gut wall into circulation. This can lead to the other organs of elimination, such as the liver and the kidneys, being put under more pressure. Now, if these organs become overwhelmed, the body will divert waste products to another elimination organ: the skin. The elimination of waste products through the skin has been linked with all manner of skin ailments from acne to eczema. Cannellini beans, like all pulses, are very high in fibre, which gives additional bulk to the stool, allowing for more regular bowel movements.

SPINACH – A wonderful source of beta-carotene, one of the most potent fat-soluble antioxidants, which can penetrate the subcutaneous layer of the skin and offer it protection against free radical damage.

PASTA WITH SPINACH AND FETA IN ROASTED RED BELL PEPPER SAUCE

SERVES 2–4

4 red bell peppers
150g wholewheat pasta
(penne works well here)
1 clove of garlic, finely
chopped
1 red onion, finely chopped
1 tablespoon olive oil, plus
extra for frying
2 handfuls of baby spinach
125g feta cheese
sea salt
side salad to serve

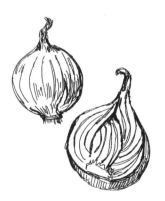

This is a great dish that screams Mediterranean sunshine, and loves your skin from within!

1. Preheat the oven to 200°C/180°C fan/400°F/gas mark 6.

2. Slice the peppers in half, remove and discard the seeds, and place them hollow side down in a baking tray, filled with about 3mm of water. Roast for 20 minutes or until the peppers have softened and the skin has started to blacken.

3. While the peppers are roasting, start boiling the pasta in a large pan of water according to the packet instructions.

4. In a separate pan, sauté the garlic and the onion in a little olive oil until the onion has softened.

5. Remove the peppers from the oven and place in a food processor. Add the garlic and onion to the food processor along with a tablespoon of olive oil and a pinch of salt. Blend into a smooth sauce, and set aside.

6. Once the pasta is cooked, drain it and add it to the pan that the onions and garlic were cooked in. Add the sauce to the pasta and mix well. Return the pan to the heat and add in the spinach. Keep stirring over the heat until the spinach has wilted.

7. Crumble over the feta cheese just before serving. Serve with a side salad.

BENEFITS

RED BELL PEPPERS – Very dense in beta-carotene and alpha-carotene, two potent members of the carotenoid family of fat-soluble antioxidants. These are the ones that migrate into the subcutaneous tissue and give antioxidant support to the collagen fibres there. Red bell peppers are also rich in a group of compounds called flavonoids. These show promise as skin-protecting compounds that deliver both antioxidant and anti-inflammatory activity.

SPINACH – A rich source of the fat-soluble antioxidant beta-carotene.

RED ONIONS – A very rich source of dietary sulphur. This mineral is vital for the production and maintenance of the extracellular matrix. This is the network of dense fibres, including collagen and elastin, which creates a great deal of structural support within tissues. The skin in particular is very dense in extracellular matrix. It requires a constant supply of sulphur to maintain itself.

FETA – The fat content of the feta will aid in the absorption of the fat-soluble compounds, so that more of them will be taken up than if they were eaten in isolation.

BALSAMIC ROASTED MEDITERRANEAN VEGETABLES WITH WHITE BEAN AND ROSEMARY MASH

SERVES 2–4

½ red bell pepper, sliced
lengthways
½ courgette, sliced lengthways
1 red onion, halved and sliced
lengthways
olive oil, for drizzling
1 tablespoon balsamic
vinegar
1 x 400g tin of cannellini
beans, drained
a sprig of fresh rosemary,
finely chopped
1 clove of garlic, finely
chopped
sea salt

This is heaven on a plate. I just love the Mediterranean influences in my diet – not only for the health benefits, but for the simple freshness of the flavours.

1. Preheat the oven to 200°C/180°C fan/400°F/gas mark 6.

2. Place the sliced vegetables in a roasting tin, and drizzle over a little olive oil and the balsamic vinegar. Add a pinch of salt and toss. Roast for about 25 minutes, stirring regularly.

3. Place the drained beans in a bowl, and mash with the back of a fork. Add a little olive oil, along with a pinch of salt and the chopped rosemary, and mix well to form a creamy mash.

4. Once the vegetables are almost cooked, sprinkle the chopped garlic over them and return to the oven for 2 minutes.

5. Remove and serve the vegetables over the mash.

BENEFITS

CANNELLINI BEANS – A rich source of the all-important B vitamins. These nutrients are involved in regulating so many processes within the skin. They regulate microcirculation to the upper and middle layers of the skin, which can help to even out skin tone. They also regulate the turnover of skin cells, plus they are vital components in the correct metabolism of essential fatty acids into their metabolic end products that deliver so many benefits.

RED BELL PEPPERS – Rich in the fat-soluble antioxidant beta-carotene. They are also very rich in a group of compounds called flavonoids. These are the phytochemicals responsible for the deep red colour. Flavonoids are by their very nature wonderful anti-inflammatories, so can be of great use in conditions such as acne and eczema. Both of these conditions feature lesions that involve a great deal of redness, which is a sign that there is active inflammation. It is therefore worthwhile to consume as many naturally anti-inflammatory compounds as possible to support healing.

RED ONIONS – Like red bell peppers, red onions are packed with flavonoids, which are responsible for that rich red-purple colour. Onions, like all of the alliums, are also very rich in organic sulphur, which helps to support the manufacture and maintenance of the extracellular matrix.

BEETROOT, RED ONION AND GOAT'S CHEESE TART

SERVES 2

olive oil, for frying
1 large red onion, thinly sliced
1 tablespoon honey
1 large sheet of readymade
  puff pastry
4 large cooked beetroot
150g goat's cheese or feta

I adore this dish. It's just heavenly, and usually when I cook it I find myself having to make more of the filling than I need to, as I munch it as I go along.

1. Add a small amount of olive oil to a large saucepan. Add the onion and sauté until it begins to soften. Add the honey and continue to cook until the onion takes on a caramelised texture.

2. Roll out the puff pastry to a size that is large enough to fit a 25cm round tart tin. Once rolled out, line the tin with the pastry and trim as necessary.

3. Preheat the oven to 200°C/180°C fan/400°F/gas mark 6. Begin by blind baking the pastry, covering it with greaseproof paper and filling with ceramic baking beads, or some dried beans.

4. Once the pastry has been blind baked for about 10 minutes, remove the baking beads and greaseproof paper. Add the caramelised onions first, ensuring the whole base of the pastry case has been covered. Then dice the cooked beetroot and sprinkle over the top of the onion layer. Lastly, crumble the cheese over the beetroot.

5. Return the tart to the oven for around 10 minutes, or until the pastry is golden brown and the cheese is softening and beginning to brown at the edges.

6. Serve with a side salad.

BENEFITS

BEETROOT – A very powerful food for liver health. Its deep-purple pigment, that stains anything and everything, is due to the phytochemical betacyanin. Betacyanin is known to be a stimulant of the phase 2 detoxification pathways in the liver. This helps to speed up and improve the way the liver deals with waste materials.

RED ONIONS – The whole allium family is rich in sulphur, which is vital to the structure and function of the extracellular matrix. Onions are also a very rich source of a prebiotic compound called inulin. This special type of sugar can be used as a food source by the good bacteria in the gut, to enhance their growth. Healthy gut flora is vital for good digestive function. If our digestive tract is healthy and we are breaking down food properly, and eliminating waste products efficiently, this will be reflected in our skin.

DESSERTS

BLACKBERRY CRUMBLE

SERVES 2–4

1 punnet of fresh blackberries
(even better if you can go
and pick them)
1 teaspoon honey
5 tablespoons porridge oats
½ teaspoon cinnamon

This is one of my absolute favourites. I have to admit, I don't have much of a sweet tooth, so often don't eat desserts. But if I'm feeling indulgent, this is a perfect example of what I'd reach for.

1. Preheat the oven to 200°C/180°C fan/400°F/gas mark 6.

2. Place the berries, honey and a tablespoon of water into a pan and simmer over a high heat. The berries will begin to break down into a mush. Keep simmering the mix until it starts to thicken.

3. Once it has started to resemble jam, transfer it to a small ovenproof dish. Top the mixture with the oats and the cinnamon, and bake for 15–20 minutes, until the oats are a golden brown.

BENEFITS

BLACKBERRIES – Very rich in a whole spectrum of antioxidants like all the dark berries. Blackberries are also packed with vitamin C, which is a vital nutrient for the manufacture of collagen.

OATS – As well as keeping the digestive system ticking along nicely thanks to their fibre content, oats are also a very rich source of the B vitamins, which help to keep the skin in peak performance and functioning at its best.

RAW KEY LIME PIE

SERVES 2–4

125g walnuts
4 tablespoons flaxseeds
5 dates, pitted and chopped
2 tablespoons coconut oil

For the filling
3 large ripe avocados
3 teaspoons honey
2 limes

This is so delicious that you will struggle to believe that it is good for so many aspects of your health, and especially for your skin. I have given this dish to hard-core junk foodies, and even they have loved it. It is a beautiful, refreshing, zesty treat.

1. To make the base, place the walnuts, flaxseeds and dates in a food processor. Gently melt 1 tablespoon of the coconut oil in a small pan on a very low temperature. Pour the melted oil into the food processor, and process to form a dough.

2. Place the dough in a pie dish, and press down evenly to cover the bottom of the dish. Place in the fridge for 2–3 hours, until set.

3. To make the filling, scoop the flesh out of the avocados into the food processor. Add the honey and the juice of both the limes, along with the zest of one of the limes.

4. Melt the remaining 1 tablespoon of coconut oil in the small pan. Pour the melted coconut oil into the food processor, and blend into a smooth purée.

5. Remove the pie base from the fridge and transfer the avocado filling into it. Return to the fridge to set. After an hour or so, the dish is ready to serve.

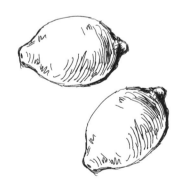

BENEFITS

AVOCADO – A wonderfully healthy food, especially for the skin. Avocados are a very rich source of the most famous fat-soluble antioxidant of them all – vitamin E! Vitamin E, due to its fat-soluble nature, will move into the subcutaneous layer of the skin and protect the structural fibres from damage, just as the carotenoids do. The unique thing about vitamin E, though, is that it can act directly on skin cells by protecting the cell membrane from being damaged by free radicals. This protection may help slow the ageing process, provided that we have a regular intake of this nutrient (let's remember how rapid the turnover of skin cells is). Avocados also contain a particular group of fats called phytosterols, which deliver huge health benefits to the cardiovascular system, and are also known to have significant anti-inflammatory activity.

As well as the above, avocados are rich in substances called polyhydroxylated fatty alcohols, which are known to assist in the absorption of compunds such as fat-soluble antioxidants!

WALNUTS – Hysteria around nuts being a supposedly 'fattening' food has luckily led to more focus on their actual benefits, and walnuts have certainly come up trumps. They are an extremely dense source of the omega 3 fatty acids that are crucial to keep the skin in tip-top condition. Walnuts are also a rich source of zinc, which helps to regulate sebum production, helps to support the immune system and aids in wound healing.

BLUEBERRY AND YOGURT LAYER CRUNCH

SERVES 1

blueberries
plain probiotic yogurt
raw porridge oats
golden flaxseeds

This is a light and virtuous dessert that's particularly great on a hot day, as it is very cooling with the yogurt and berries together.

You will notice that I haven't put specific weights or amounts for these ingredients. It's literally a case of having the ingredients handy, and creating the recipe in layers according to the size of your serving vessel.

1. Start with a layer of blueberries.

2. On top of the blueberries place a layer of yogurt, then a layer of oats, then a layer of flaxseeds.

3. Repeat this process until your serving vessel is full.

BENEFITS

BLUEBERRIES – Blueberries are packed with a broad range of antioxidant compounds, such as flavonoids. They're also rich in vitamin C, which is a vital nutrient for the manufacture of collagen.

FLAXSEEDS – These luscious crunchy seeds are full of omega 3 fatty acids. Inflammation-busting, skin-softening and all-round health-improvers!

OATS – A great source of the B vitamins. Remember, these nutrients are involved, at one stage or another, in regulating almost every physiological process in the skin, whether it's circulation, or skin cell turnover, or even wound healing and oil secretion. Any food source that offers good levels of these nutrients will help the skin to function better as a whole.

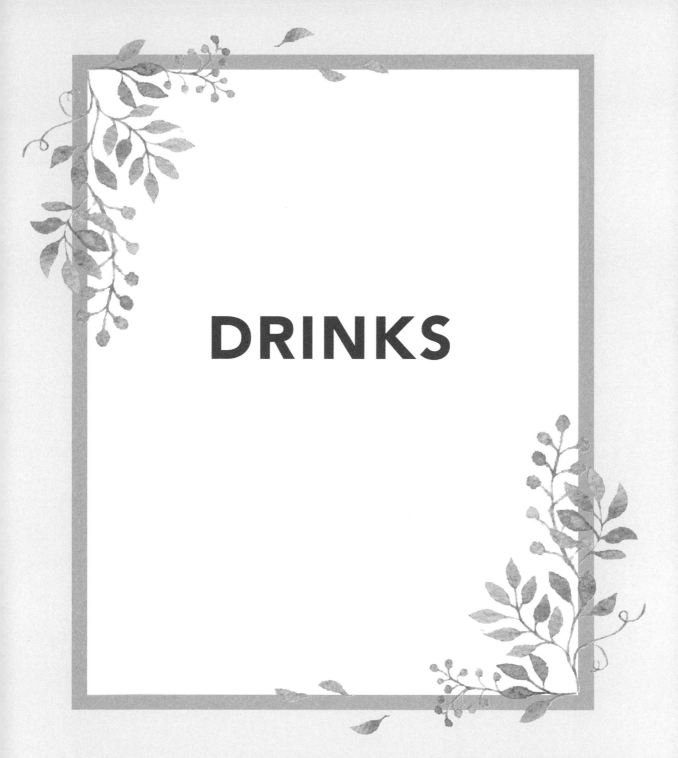

DRINKS

A NOTE ABOUT THESE RECIPES:

These recipes will generally require a juicer and/or a blender. If you have never tried making your own juices at home, then it really is worth having a go. It used to be a laborious and messy affair, but modern juicers make it an absolute breeze, and they are a doddle to clean. The beauty of juices is that you get a huge amount of nutrition without having to plough your way through a ton of fresh fruit and veg. It is also worth investing in a decent blender.

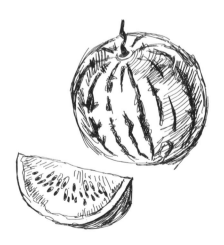

SKIN TONIC TEA

SERVES 1–2

2 teaspoons dried red clover
2 teaspoons dandelion leaf
2 teaspoons cleavers
2 teaspoons calendula

OK, I couldn't resist it. As I am a medical herbalist, I thought it only right that I should use some of these wonderful medicinal tools in this book. Dried herbs are easy to obtain, and herbal teas are wonderful to sip on throughout the day. Don't underestimate the power of a tea, though. Much of the active chemistry in medicinal plants will be water-soluble, and something as simple as an infusion will create a powerful phytochemical cocktail. I usually brew my teas in a medium-sized cafetiere. All of these herbs are freely available at a reputable herbal supplier (see useful contacts section).

Now, I hope you are paying attention . . . simply add all the herbs to the pot, and cover with hot water! Steep for about 10–15 minutes before drinking.

BENEFITS

RED CLOVER – Red clover is one of my favourite skin herbs. It seems to have the amazing ability to reduce the movement of waste products through the skin. In our modern world, it is the norm for our bodies to be bombarded with challenging compounds that put a strain on our organs of elimination such as the liver and kidneys. When these are already hard at work, the body will start to look at other ways to get rid of waste products, and one of these ways is through the skin. This can be a trigger for some skin conditions to flare up or worsen.

DANDELION LEAF – Dandelion leaves are a very powerful natural diuretic. This means that they stimulate the kidneys to increase urinary output. This helps the kidneys to remove water-soluble waste products more quickly, reducing the likelihood that waste products are sent to the skin for removal.

CLEAVERS – Cleavers, otherwise known as goose grass or sticky willy, is a very powerful herb for cleansing the lymphatic system. The lymphatic system is like a second circulatory system that drains waste products from the tissues. Cells eject their waste products into the lymphatic fluid that bathes them. This fluid then makes its way to the lymphatic vessels, and eventually to the blood for waste removal via the kidneys. The movement of lymphatic fluid around the body is dependent on muscular contractions to squeeze it along. This can sometimes mean that it takes a while for waste products to reach the kidneys. Cleavers contain a group of chemicals called coumarins (these are the same chemicals you smell with freshly cut grass). These compounds cause the walls of the lymphatic vessels to contract. This contraction increases the pressure within the vessel. When the pressure increases the lymphatic fluid is moved along more easily, which, in short, will lead to faster removal of waste products – again, lessening the risk of waste products being routed through the skin.

CALENDULA – Calendula has a long history of being a powerful herb for skin health. The bright-orange colour pigments in the flower petals are effective anti-inflammatory agents, and have traditionally been used during skin flare-ups for centuries. Calendula, like cleavers, is also a great lymphatic tonic, helping to keep this system clean.

RASPBERRY AND MELON COOLER

SERVES 1

150g fresh raspberries
½ watermelon
1 apple
sparkling mineral water

This is such a delicious drink, and served in a cool glass on a hot day it can make you feel like you're relaxing on the beach. Nice!

1. Run all the ingredients through a juicer, except the sparkling water.

2. When serving, fill a glass two-thirds with juice, and then top up with sparkling water.

BENEFITS

RASPBERRIES – Raspberries are a wonderful source of vitamin C and, when consumed in their raw state as they are here, the vitamin C levels will remain intact. Vitamin C is a vitally important factor for the production of collagen. So, if you want to keep skin looking young and healthy, a consistently high intake of vitamin C is essential.

WATERMELON – Watermelons are high in several important skin nutrients. Like raspberries they are a rich source of vitamin C for collagen support. They are also very high in beta-carotene, that champion of fat-soluble antioxidants.

GREEN SMOOTHIE

SERVES 1

1 banana
a handful of red grapes
2 large handfuls of baby
  spinach leaves
200ml apple juice

This recipe is an absolute winner! I have made this smoothie on numerous radio and TV shows, often to the disbelief of the presenters. They look at what goes into it, and the colour of it, and are shocked when they actually taste it and love every drop. It contains loads of greens, but all you can taste is the fruit. You will be shocked too!

Blend all the ingredients in a blender and enjoy!

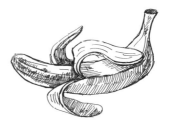

BENEFITS

SPINACH – Huge amounts of beta-carotene, plus vitamin C and anti-inflammatory compounds such as flavonoids. Spinach is also rich in minerals including zinc.

RED GRAPES – Red grapes are a rich source of collagen-boosting vitamin C. They are also host to a very broad spectrum of antioxidants, most notably the heart-healthy anthocyanins, which are members of the flavonoid family.

CARROT, APPLE, BEETROOT AND CELERY JUICE

SERVES 1

1 large carrot
1 large apple
1 small beetroot
2 sticks of celery

This deep-coloured juice is incredibly potent, and very tasty. The sweetness of the apple really comes through and disguises the fact that there are veggies in it.

Simply run all the ingredients through a juicer.

BENEFITS

CARROTS – Carrots are a very dense source of beta-carotene, the plant form of vitamin A, and the most powerful of the carotenoids – those fat-soluble anti-oxidants. Just to give you an idea of how well these compounds accumulate in the subcutaneous layer of the skin, there is a condition called hypercarotenemia. This is where the skin of people who eat a lot of carrots will actually turn orange due to the sheer level of carotenoids that have accumulated there. That's proof!

APPLES – Apples have a high vitamin C content, and also contain a powerful chemical called ellagic acid. This has well-documented antioxidant properties and has been shown to be an effective liver stimulant, helping in the detoxification process.

BEETROOT – Beetroot also has a powerful effect on liver function. The deep-purple colour pigment so characteristic of this vegetable influences phase 2 detoxification in the liver, which can help to keep things on the inside clean.

CELERY – Celery is a very rich source of so many minerals, including potassium, sodium and magnesium. These minerals help to keep the body hydrated. There is nothing worse for the overall appearance of the skin than dehydration. The minerals in celery make this juice very hydrating. Interestingly, there is a dichotomy here as celery also has a mild diuretic effect, meaning it increases urinary output. It has the ability to make the kidneys work a little harder, but without overdoing it to the point where someone would get dehydrated.

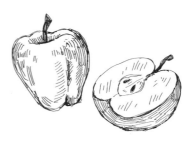

SPINACH, CUCUMBER AND CANTALOUPE MELON JUICE

SERVES 1

2 handfuls of baby spinach
½ cucumber
cantaloupe melon

This is an amazing tasting juice. Sweet, fragrant, divine. Not to mention the nutrient density it contains.

Run all the ingredients through a juicer. Put the spinach leaves in first and use the other ingredients to push them through.

BENEFITS

CUCUMBER – Cucumbers are surprisingly nutrient-dense. They contain vitamin C and some minerals, the most interesting of which is silica. This is the mineral responsible for the luscious shiny skin of the cucumber. Silica is a vital component in the manufacture of collagen and the maintenance of its flexibility, helping the skin to become more resilient to sagging and wrinkling.

CANTALOUPE MELON – This is included in this juice for two main reasons. Firstly, its flavour complements that of cucumber beautifully. Secondly, and most importantly, it is a very rich source of carotenoids, those fat-soluble antioxidants. There is also a reasonable amount of vitamin C in cantaloupes too.

SPINACH – Spinach is another rich source of vitamin C. Gram for gram it has more vitamin C than an orange! There is also, of course, a huge dose of beta-carotene in spinach leaves, making this juice a fat-soluble antioxidant bath for your skin.

THE VIRIDIAN CLEAR SKIN PROJECT

Before I sign off, I wanted to give a nod towards Viridian Nutrition, a supplement company I occasionally work with. Viridian's supplements complement what I want to do for my clients – get them the nutrients they need to make their skin as healthy and glowy as it should be. So together we set up the Clear Skin Project, where 47 people cooked my recipes while taking Viridian supplements: two Clear Skin Complex capsules and three teaspoons of Clear Skin Omega Oil at breakfast each day. The results were incredible: 76 per cent of people found their skin was better after 60 days of taking part. Here are a couple of those success stories, and see the Resources section on page 157 for more information about Viridian.

BEFORE AFTER

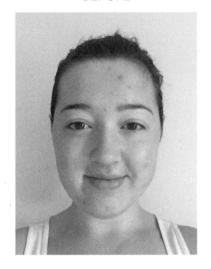 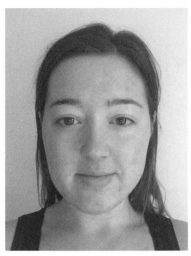

LUCY – age 25

Why did you apply for the Clear Skin Project and what were you looking to achieve?

I am a huge fan of Viridian's products and ethos and knew of their beauty range, so when I saw their Clear Skin Project on Twitter in association with Dale Pinnock, I replied immediately. I was looking to achieve a better complexion and reduce spots and redness.

How did you feel in yourself before taking part?

Unconfident – people would notice my bad skin and make comments on it. I was frustrated because I felt my diet was generally good and yet my skin didn't reflect that.

How did you feel after taking part?

The fact that other people are commenting on how great my skin looks says it all! Even after the first two weeks of this programme I noticed improvements with less spots and more moisture in my skin. My confidence has massively improved and I am now comfortable wearing less make-up too. An added benefit is my hair feels stronger, softer and shinier!

What were your favourite recipes?

The soups – I found them very nourishing and satisfying. I also loved the Moroccan-style Veggie Tagine and Thai Prawn Curry, and in general found all the recipes easy to make and also easy to adapt depending on what ingredients I had in the fridge e.g. adding sweet potato or fish to a curry.

BEFORE

AFTER

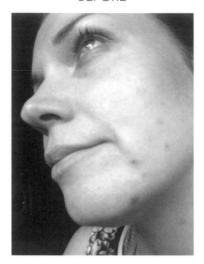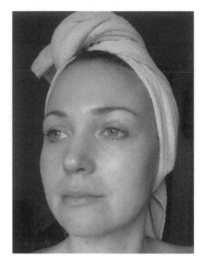

OLIVIA – age 35

Why did you apply for the Clear Skin Project and what were you looking to achieve?

I've had blemished, unbalanced, problem skin ever since my teenage years. I have tried many different topical skin products but working from within has been a much better approach to helping my skin improve – and it has been easy to incorporate both the supplements and the recipes into my daily life.

How did you feel in yourself before taking part?

I wasn't 100% happy with my skin and I wanted to make changes to benefit it and give it extra longevity.

How did you feel after taking part?

My skin feels a little smoother and I have definitely noticed a more even skin tone; no red blotches on my face anymore.

What were your favourite recipes?

I found all the recipes to be no hassle; there are only a handful of ingredients for each and they are easy to prepare. I cooked the Proper Bell Pepper Soup and the Pasta with Spinach and Feta the most, as they are very family-friendly. I don't buy soft drinks, so we also enjoyed the juices and smoothie recipes, which are a delicious way of getting fresh nutrient rich goodness into my children.

RECIPE INDEX

GENERAL INDEX

R
riboflavin, *see* vitamin B2
rosacea 55–7
    foods to counter 57
    nutrients to counter 56

S
selenium 22, 32, 46, 52
silica 33
skin 10, *see also* dermis, epidermis, minerals,
        nutrients, subcutis, vitamins
    ageing 16–19, *see also* free radicals
    as a sensory organ 12
    disorders 20–2, *see also individual entries*
    flushing 55
    function of 11
    and immune system 11
    producing vitamin D 12
    regulating temperature 11–12
    structure of 12–15, *see also* dermis,
        epidermis, subcutis
    temperature and microcapillaries 14
subcutis 14–15, 38, 39
    ageing of 18
sugar 31

sulphur 33
sweat glands 12, 14

T
testosterone 33
thiamin see vitamin B1

V
vitamins, and skincare 23–9
    preserved in cooking 29
    A 25, 38, 45, 51
    the B vitamins 29, 49, 51, 54, 56
    B 25–6
    B1 26
    B2 26
    B3 26–7
    B5 27
    B6 27
    B12 28, 29
    C 21, 28, 29, 45, 46
    D 12, 28, 55
    E 22, 29, 38

Z
zinc 21, 33–4, 45–6

RESOURCES

British Dietetic Association
Articles, news, research, guidance and fact sheets
around all aspects of nutrition and health.
www.bda.uk.com

British Nutrition Foundation
An extensive resource for all things nutrition.
Articles, research summaries, publications and more.
www.nutrition.org.uk

British Skin Foundation
Latest research, articles, tips and fundraising events.
www.britishskinfoundation.org.uk

National Eczema Society
Support, self-care and management advice,
latest research and interesting articles.
www.eczema.org

Viridian Nutrition
An extensive range of the cleanest supplements around.
More than 200+ products including vitamins, minerals, herbs,
oils and specialist formulae made using the purest ingredients,
with absolutely no additives, nasty fillers or junk.
www.viridian-nutrition.com

ABOUT THE AUTHOR

DALE PINNOCK is a renowned nutritionist, medical herbalist, chef and health expert with a burning interest in the way that food can be a powerful medicine. His passion is explaining to people, in a practical, fun and exciting way, how to easily make sense of the barrage of information about how food affects their health. He is a regular on television, radio and in the press, spreading this message far and wide. Dale qualified in both Nutrition and Herbal Medicine and trained at the University of Westminster. He runs private healthcare clinics in Cambridgeshire and Hertfordshire where he combines herbal medicine with nutritional healing to provide a full and far-reaching therapeutic programme.

This edition first published in Great Britain in 2018
by Orion Publishing Group Ltd
Carmelite House, 50 Victoria Embankment
London EC4Y 0DZ
An Hachette UK Company

1 3 5 7 9 10 8 6 4 2

A CIP catalogue record for this book
is available from the British Library.

ISBN: 9781409166382

Illustrations: Shutterstock

Printed in Italy

This is an update of *The Clear Skin Cookbook*,
first published by Constable & Robinson in 2012

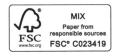

www.orionbooks.co.uk